EIGHT WEEKS TO OPTIMUM HEALTH

EIGHT WEEKS TO OPTIMUM HEALTH

A Proven Program for Taking
Full Advantage of Your Body's
Natural Healing Power

ANDREW WEIL, M.D.

Alfred A. Knopf NEW YORK 1997

THIS IS A BORZOI BOOK
PUBLISHED BY ALFRED A. KNOPF, INC.

Grateful acknowledgment is made to the following for permission to reprint previously published material:

Beacon Press: Excerpts from *The Miracle of Mindfulness: A Manual on Meditation* by Thich Nhat Hanh, translated by Mobi Ho, copyright © 1975, 1976 by Thich Nhat Hanh. Reprinted by permission of Beacon Press.

Doubleday: "A Forgiveness Meditation" from *Healing into Life and Death* by Stephen Levine, copyright © 1987 by Stephen Levine. Reprinted by permission of Doubleday Dell Publishing Group, Inc.

The Office of Tibet: Excerpt from the Nobel Peace Prize acceptance speech of His Holiness the Dalai Lama (1989). Reprinted by permission of The Office of Tibet on behalf of The Office of His Holiness the Dalai Lama, Dharamsala.

Library of Congress Cataloging-in-Publication Data
Weil, Andrew.
Eight weeks to optimum health / Andrew Weil.
p.   cm.
Includes bibliographical references and index.
ISBN 0-679-44715-6 (alk. paper)
1. Self-care, health.   2. Alternative medicine.   3. Health behavior.   I. Title.
RA776.95.W45   1997
613—dc21   96-51918
CIP

Manufactured in the United States of America
PUBLISHED MARCH 14, 1997
REPRINTED FOUR TIMES
SIXTH PRINTING, APRIL 1997

CONTENTS

Part One

THE CAPACITY
TO CHANGE

1

PEOPLE CAN CHANGE

YOU HAVE IN YOUR HANDS a tool for changing your life, an Eight-Week Program for improving health and gaining access to the power of spontaneous healing in your body. I will guide you through this program step by step, explaining the changes I will ask you to make in how you eat, how you exercise, how you breathe, and how you use your mind. I will recommend vitamins, minerals, and herbs you can use to protect your body's healing system, and I will give you ideas about how you can change long-standing patterns of behavior that impair optimal health.

Maybe you have picked up this book because you want to have more energy. Maybe you want to lose some weight. Maybe you worry about getting older and developing diseases that disabled your parents. Perhaps you travel frequently and find it hard to maintain a healthy lifestyle on the road. Or perhaps you have a chronic illness, minor or major, and want to be less dependent on pharmaceutical drugs. Regardless of the specific nature of your need or concern, the information I have assembled in these pages will help you draw on your body's own resources for natural healing.

The Eight-Week Program consists of small steps that build on each other until, by the time you complete it, you have laid the foundation for healthy living. You can then decide how much of the program you want to maintain on a permanent basis. I assume that you want to make changes in your life—otherwise you wouldn't be reading this book. I see my job as pointing you in the right direction. I have no doubt that you can change, because I know from my own experience that people can do so if they really want to.

In moving files recently, I came across a yellowed clipping from *The New York Times* of August 12, 1971, with the headline: "Meat-Eating 230-Pound Doctor Is Now 175-Pound Vegetarian." The article was the featured story in the Food–Fashions–Family Furnishings section of that day's paper and carried the byline of Raymond A. Sokolov, then a *Times* food writer. It concerns a twenty-nine-year-old physician in rural Virginia who gave up animal foods except for dairy products, with a resultant increase in energy, well-being, and overall health. There is a photograph of the doctor in his kitchen preparing fresh corn. He has a full black beard, is wearing blue jeans and a work shirt, and looks content. Next to the picture is his recipe for a rich corn soup containing milk and butter, and another recipe for a barley-and-vegetable casserole that calls for a quarter-cup of peanut oil. According to the article, the doctor's interest in consciousness led him to experiment with yoga and meditation, and "since yoga calls for a vegetarian diet, he gave up meat 'in order to really do it right.' He has been vegetarian ever since, to the amazement of his friends, who remember him as a voracious meat eater and a fat person while at Harvard. . . . In one year on his new diet [he] has reduced from 230 to 175 pounds. His recurring colds and allergies have vanished. . . ."

My beard is no longer black, and I have not been able to maintain my weight at 175 pounds. I am still mostly vegetarian (I have eaten fish for the past ten years), though now I don't make rich soups with milk and butter, use oil in such quantities, or ever cook with peanut oil. I think I am wiser with age and in general feel much happier now than I did when I was twenty-nine.

That was a watershed year for me. I had quit a frustrating job with the National Institute of Mental Health in July 1970, dropped out of professional medicine to write my first book, and made a great many changes in my way of living besides giving up meat. For the first time ever, I lived alone in a natural setting well away from a city. I had no office to go to, no obligations to meet. I began each morning with sitting meditation for as long as I could tolerate, which was not much in those days. I took long walks in the woods, practiced yoga postures in the afternoons, wrote, and read on a variety of subjects that interested me, from Native American shamanism to mushrooms and other wild foods. By August 1971, I was nearing another transition.

The *New York Times* article noted, "Dr. Weil will be traveling to the Amazon jungle this fall for an extended visit to some primitive tribes on a fellowship from the Institute of Current World Affairs, a New York foundation."

I held that fellowship from 1971 to 1975 and have written elsewhere about those travels. In my recent book, *Spontaneous Healing*, I describe seeking out a shaman in Colombia during that period and explain that my studies of ethnobotany and medicine at Harvard made me want to see the rain forest, meet native healers, and try to understand the source of healing. Mostly I wanted to learn how to help people get well and stay well without using so many of the invasive and suppressive methods of conventional medicine, and I thought the knowledge I needed was to be found in remote mountains and jungles, far from classrooms and clinics. My plan was to go to southern Mexico to learn Spanish, then to make my way down to Colombia, Ecuador, and Peru to live with Indians and learn their ways with plants and healing.

I knew this journey would be demanding, and when I first settled on the idea, I was in no way prepared, either physically or mentally, to undertake such an adventure. I had grown up in a row house in Philadelphia with little opportunity to spend time in nature, let alone in wilderness. On leaving Philadelphia, I attended college and medical school in Boston, then completed a medical internship in San Francisco—more urban, indoor experience. I was not very comfortable out-of-doors, being nervous about insects and wary of the sun, since I had fair skin that never tanned, only burned; I accepted this as an inherited trait that could never disappear. Although I was able to concentrate enough to handle schoolwork easily, I was restless, very susceptible to boredom, and I craved distraction. I was largely sedentary, hating exercise, and since I also liked to eat, I was overweight. My diet was free-form and thoughtless. I ate anything and everything in large quantities, including very high-fat foods. I was a frequent consumer of alcohol and Coca-Cola.

Though I had no significant health problems, I knew from the way I huffed and puffed climbing stairs that I was not in good cardiovascular condition. I suffered from intense pollen allergies, mostly in the summer, and also had allergic reactions to a number of medications and some foods. Sometimes I would get hives for no apparent reason. On occasion I got bad migraines.

So it was clear that I was going to have to change in order to set out by myself for unknown lands and peoples in the Andes and the Amazon basin. Many of my friends could not imagine my doing any such thing, but I was determined to do so, because I believed it was the only way for me to become a true physician, one who could work with the healing power of nature. When I think back on all the changes I made in the year before I left the United States, I do not remember their being hard, even though I had to give up lifelong habits and adopt new ways of being. My memories of that year are of much fun and discovery along with a gratifying sense of accomplishment. When I look at before and after pictures of myself, I am amazed at the difference. Not only did I lose weight and grow a beard, I became aware of my strength and flexibility, got much more comfortable with myself and nature, and even, miraculously, was able to stay out in the sun and tan for the first time in my life. My allergies and headaches disappeared. By the time I got to southern Mexico, I was feeling better than I ever had in my life, full of energy, ready to plunge into unknown waters.

My late friend and mentor, Norman Zinberg, a Harvard psychoanalyst, used to keep that photo of me from *The New York Times*— and a more recent photo—to refute those who complained to him that people could not change, and change permanently. His profession was about helping patients give up dysfunctional patterns of thought and behavior, not an easy job. As a physician and health counselor today, I find myself in the same position. Patients come to me with stories of woe, and instead of giving them magical cures, I tell them they must change their diets, their habits of exercise, their ways of handling stress, even their breathing. Fortunately, the patients who come to me are self-selected. They share my philosophy of health and healing and are highly motivated to take responsibility for their well-being. They are looking for advice about what to do, and when they get it, they will act on it. Unfortunately, most doctors deal with patients who are not so motivated and are instead looking for quick fixes, who would rather take a prescribed drug than change their behavior.

But I know from my experience as a physician that many of the common complaints that people have these days respond much better to simple adjustments of lifestyle than to taking medicine. You can certainly medicate yourself regularly with painkillers if you are prone to headaches, or with antihistamines if you have allergies, anti-inflammatories if you have arthritis, or sedatives if you can't sleep, but how much better it would be to solve those problems by modifying diet and patterns of activity and rest and by using natural remedies. The Eight-Week Program presented in this book gives you all the information you need to do that and more. Above all, it will enhance and protect your body's own healing system, which is your best defense against illness, the stress of modern life, and the assaults of a toxic environment.

I do not mean to minimize the difficulty of change. *Inertia* is resistance to motion, action, or change. Just as physical bodies at rest tend to remain at rest, whereas those in motion tend to remain in motion in straight lines unless acted upon by external forces, so do human bodies resist change. Inertia is a general characteristic of things both living and nonliving. If you have ever tried to work a block of cold modeling clay or a lump of unkneaded bread dough, you know the persistence and effort required to make them flowing and supple. In these cases the external force comes from skilled hands, experienced at working clay and dough and overcoming their inertia.

Many people want to remake their lives but cannot imagine doing so without outside help. If only some skilled hands could apply the necessary force to get them going, they could do it, but on their own they remain in habitual ruts. The answer to this common problem is motivation. The very word derives from the Latin form of the verb "to move." If you are motivated to seek better health, all that you need to achieve it is practical information. The Eight-Week Program is complete and sufficient for you to reach your goal. If you are motivated to read this book and begin the program, you need no other outside help.

Let me share with you some observations about the power of motivation to break even the most stubborn of unhealthy habits—drug addiction. Over the years, I have worked with many people who struggled with addictive behavior: smokers, drinkers, compulsive users of cocaine, heroin, coffee, and chocolate (as well as compulsive eaters, gamblers, and shoppers). I have learned that any addiction can be broken if people are motivated to do so. Even addiction to a substance like heroin, a "hard" drug, drops away easily when users develop sufficient motivation to stop. The trouble, of course, is that therapists and programs cannot put motivation into addicts, and many addicts who check themselves into programs or go to therapists do not really want to stop, no matter what they say.

Tobacco addiction is the most common cause of preventable, serious illness in our society. As a physician I am often in the position of trying to convince smokers that they must attempt to break their addiction; as a longtime researcher of drugs and drug abuse, I know that cigarettes are the most addictive substance in the world. Nonetheless, I have known many people to quit successfully and permanently. How do they do it?

Many ex-smokers made one or more unsuccessful attempts to quit before they finally did it for good. Some describe intense physical and psychological distress during their early attempts but report that when they finally kicked the habit there was no struggle. One man told me he woke up one day, reached for his first cigarette of the morning, and suddenly saw his stained fingers and the dirty ashtray as if for the first time. In that moment he realized he had had enough. He quit without difficulty and has never smoked since. "Once I had that realization, it was easy," he remembers. "I knew I would never smoke again."

What do these stories tell us about the possibility of changing behavior? My interpretation of them is that motivation is the key: when it reaches a critical point, breaking even the hardest of drug addictions can be easy. How motivation develops to that point is not simple or obvious.

Research into cigarette addiction indicates that making an attempt to quit is the best predictor of eventual success, even if the attempt itself is not successful. For this reason, I always ask smokers who come to see me whether they have ever made an attempt to quit, and always urge them to set a date when they will make one. Attempting to quit is commitment to changing behavior, a measure of motivation, and whether you succeed or fail is less important than making the attempt. Even if you resume smoking in a week, you lose no credit for the effort. In fact, the effort adds to a reservoir of motivation that one day will be full enough to initiate the sudden change that enables people to drop habits without struggling. Such is the power of motivation, but it must come from within. Whether you are a therapist, counselor, friend, or relative of an addict, all you can do is give good reasons for changing behavior along with encouragement and support.

This book is all about changing behavior. You are probably not addicted to drugs, but you may have other habits that are keeping you from experiencing optimum health and raising your risks of disease. Perhaps you like high-fat foods and eat no vegetables, or never exercise, or drink too much coffee, or have unsatisfying relationships, or live with anxiety or depression. You can change your behavior in ways that will protect and enhance your body's natural healing ability, and from the fact that you are reading this book, I know that you already are motivated to do so.

When I was a sedentary, overweight, allergic person who craved distraction and was uncomfortable in nature, I was able to alter my way of being completely and relatively easily because *I wanted very much to do something that required me to change.* I knew that I could not undertake the journey to South America as I was; it was my desire to make the trip that inspired me to work on myself, and that desire outweighed the benefits I was getting from my established patterns of living.

This is an important point. If you simply condemn unwanted behavior without acknowledging what you are getting out of it, you may not be able to give it up no matter how much harm it is causing. In order to change behavior, you must be clear about what satisfaction that behavior is giving you as well as what it is costing you, then make a conscious decision to move. Again take the example of smoking. It is very easy to see it only as a dirty, unhealthy habit with nothing to recommend it, but for a smoker cigarettes provide pleasure, relief from nervous tension, improved concentration, and feelings of well-being, even if temporary. One woman who was still in the phase of struggling with her addiction put it this way: "Cigarettes are my friends—or, I should say, they are more like lovers. My relationship with them is deeply intimate, and the thought of never having them again desolates me just as if I were never to see a lover again." Becoming a nonsmoker would have to offer a great reward indeed to compensate her for that loss.

Now, it is obvious that fear can be a great motivator. The threat of imminent death can make people quit smoking readily, no matter that cigarettes are their "friends" and "lovers." The possibility of divorce can lead spouses finally to spend more quality time with each other. Fear of flunking out of college may motivate a student to buckle down and study. So avoidance of disaster may be more than adequate compensation for giving up a beloved habit or long-established pattern of behavior. In the example I gave from my own history, however, the reward was not avoidance of a negative outcome but, rather, enjoyment of a positive one: I got to go on my Latin American adventures and have wonderful experiences that I would not trade for anything.

Even though I recognize the efficacy of fear in facilitating behavioral change, I feel that seeking positive reinforcement (a reward you can enjoy) is better than pursuing negative reinforcement (avoidance of something you do not want to experience), because research shows that positive reinforcement is better at *maintaining* new behavior. If fear is your motivator, when fear subsides, so does motivation. Fear can also paralyze you, preventing you from moving at all. I promise that I will not try to scare you into following my Eight-Week Program. Instead I will describe the real rewards that await you on completing it and making it a part of your life.

You will notice that I will not ask you to give up many things. I will not ask you to stop eating meat or drinking coffee or alcohol, or even say a word about quitting smoking. You will not have to give up sex or chocolate on this program either. All I will ask you to do is to add positive behaviors, to strengthen and extend habits you probably already have, habits of eating, exercising, breathing, using your mind, and nourishing your spirit. I will leave it to you to moderate or eliminate any unhealthy behavior. As you become more aware of your body's healing system and your responsibility for protecting it, I think that will happen naturally, without forcing change.

To reinforce the point that people can change, I'd like to quote from letters I have received. Here first is T.J. from Minnesota:

Six years ago (I'm now twenty-seven) the doctors threw the ugly "C-word" at me and made it sound like a death sentence. (It was bone cancer.) They decided that they were the authorities and I was the victim and the only way was their way. I walked out of their offices never to return. I took up biking (about five hundred miles a week) and running (about sixty miles a week), and ate fresh fruit, juices, and whole grains . . . nothing else. Too bad more people out there won't acknowledge what a little self-determination and using one's subconscious can do to return a person to wholeness. I'm graduating in six weeks with a B.Sc. in exercise science and physiology and my minor in psychology. I hope to work toward developing programs for others to offer them alternative pathways toward health and wholeness. It was an inspiration to know that there are some doctors who believe that healing can come from within and not merely from them. Just how far is it from Minnesota to Arizona? I think I'll bike out there after graduation to live in a climate my joints will like a little better.

The next letter is from Barbara Levy Daniels, a counselor from Williamsville, New York:

I am a fifty-year-old healthy female who has been seeking medical advice for a rheumatoidlike condition for the past twelve years. With each attempt, Western doctors told me I had rheumatoid arthritis and that the most conservative treatment was anti-inflammatory medications. These did nothing to relieve my swollen joints or my intense fatigue.

It became apparent to me over the years that most doctors had no idea how to help me other than to give out medicines. They never asked me about diet, vitamins, or exercise.

Now I have eliminated dairy products, artificial sweeteners, caffeine, and acidic fruits and eat a vegetarian diet. I have followed your simple vitamin formula and have had several acupuncture treatments. I have continued daily exercise and have a massage from a massage therapist about once a month.

I have followed this routine for approximately five months and find myself much improved. The morning fatigue is mostly gone as is the multiple joint pain. I feel like my "old" self again.

If more doctors practiced in this way, the costs of health care could be reduced.

And this from Shelley Griffith of Massena, New York:

I was on a program of my own due to the tragic (suicide) death of my twenty-year-old son, which took my health down the tubes. Then I ran across your book when I was searching for advice to bring my physical body back to good alignment. Bingo! (I was going to a standard practitioner, by the way, and I am never going back.) Your consciousness-raising methods are so ahead of Western, sterile, nonspiritual methodology, anyone with any sense of the greater picture will take heed. So—I started going to places with spiritual energy: went on retreats, visited shrines, did healing ceremonies. This brought me the ability to give up my pain that had soaked deeply into my physical body. I needed the Eight-Week Program to get rid of accumulated toxicity. I brought flowers indoors, did away with all vegetable oils, brought in extra-virgin olive oil, worked with garlic (excellent and easy for me, because I'm Italian-French). And I went to the health-food store for organic flours, grains, and beans. I decreased animal protein and bought green tea. I take echinacea and practice news fasts. My personal development has been super, with renewed energy. The deep breathing has almost eliminated the grief, pain, and anxiety. Depression has lessened considerably, my weight has dropped, my chest pain has disappeared, and my circulatory system is back in balance. I also take some of the tonics you recommend, especially ginger and dong quai. I'm learning all I can.

I will try to accomplish three things in the pages that follow. First, I want to share with you my vision of the body's healing system and encourage you to rely on it in all matters concerning your health. Second, I want to convince you of the importance of developing a healthy lifestyle and the possibility of doing so quickly and easily. Third, I want to give you very specific suggestions about those aspects of lifestyle that I consider most important to health and healing. I know that I cannot motivate you to undertake the Eight-Week Program—you must do that yourself—but since you have read this far, I believe you are already interested in moving forward, and I will assume that you now want to know what moving forward entails and how to do it.

2

An Overview of Health and Healing

HEALTH IS WHOLENESS AND BALANCE, an inner resilience that allows you to meet the demands of living without being overwhelmed. If you have that kind of resilience, you can experience the inevitable interactions with germs and not get infections, you can be in contact with allergens and not suffer allergies, and you can sustain exposure to carcinogens and not get cancer. Optimal health should also bring with it a sense of strength and joy, so that you experience it as more than just the absence of disease. I designed the Eight-Week Program to lead you to that experience and show you how to maintain it.

Perfect health is not possible: beware of persons and products that promise it. Health is a dynamic and temporary state of equilibrium destined to break down as conditions change, but most of the breakdowns need not be major. The point is that health is not static; it is normal to lose it periodically in order to come back to it in a better way. Whenever the equilibrium of the body breaks down, your healing system attempts to re-establish it. In other words, healing is an automatic process activated by any breakdown in health. When you cut your finger, for example, you do not have to pray for the cut to heal or seek out a finger healer. As long as the wound is clean, and no underlying chronic illness is present, the cut heals by itself. That is an example of *spontaneous healing*, mediated by the healing system.

The *healing system* is a functional system of the body, not a structural component like the nervous system or the musculoskeletal system. Western medicine focuses more on structure than on function, with the result that conventional doctors learn a great deal about the body's structural systems and less about functional ones. Of course, in some cases—digestion and circulation, for example—structure and function are synonymous, but because the healing system does not correlate neatly with any one set of body structures, I cannot provide a line drawing of the healing system in the way that I could of the digestive system. The function of healing depends on the operation of all the systems known to Western medicine; it also draws on the mind and other nonphysical components of our beings.

To see the difference between looking at the body as a set of associated structures versus a set of interdependent functions, it is instructive to contrast Eastern medical science with Western. Traditional Chinese medicine developed thousands of years ago in a sophisticated culture that pioneered the discovery and orderly use of medicinal plants and invented a unique therapeutic modality—acupuncture—that is now widely practiced throughout the world. For a variety of cultural reasons—one being the unthinkability of dissecting a dead body—Chinese medicine also developed without detailed knowledge of the internal structure of the human body. Instead, it concentrated on identifying body functions and clarifying their relationships to each other.

One key function, identified long ago by Eastern medical science, is *defense*—that is, the body has the need and ability to defend itself against threats to its equilibrium, whether they be physical, emotional, or energetic. Having noted and studied the body's defensive capabilities, Chinese doctors then explored the natural world to find ways of maintaining and enhancing them, and they discovered a number of ways to do so, including the administration of herbal remedies. Among these remedies are ginseng, astragalus, and several mushrooms that grow on trees, such as *Ganoderma lucidum* (known to the Chinese as *ling chih* and the Japanese as *reishi*).

Chinese doctors knew little of the nature of the organs that Western medicine now considers parts of the immune systems; they did not connect tonsils, adenoids, the lymph nodes, appendix, thymus, and spleen with the body's defensive sphere of function; but that lack of anatomical knowledge did not obstruct their practical ability to improve the health of their patients. On the other hand, Western doctors described the structural nature of the immune organs but had no idea of their function until very recently; for much of this century, they labeled most of them "functionless," "vestigial," or "unimportant." Even when I was a student at Harvard Medical School in the late 1960s, it was commonplace for surgeons to remove tonsils and adenoids from most children who had frequent episodes of tonsillitis. Until very recently, many patients who entered hospitals for abdominal surgery—gall-bladder removals or hysterectomies, for example—had their appendixes removed routinely and without their consent, often not finding out that removals had taken place until they got their hospital bills.

In the 1950s, doctors in leading medical centers recklessly injured the thymus glands of children with X-rays. They invented a disease, thymic hypertrophy, that every child had, curable by shrinking the gland with X-ray treatments. A hypertrophic organ is one that is too large. The thymus is large in childhood because it is doing vital work for the developing immune system: programming lymphocytes to recognize foreign antigens. Doctors in the 1950s did not understand that function. They believed the thymus was a useless organ, whose large size in childhood indicated some disease process.

Here is a stark contrast between a functional versus a structural view of the human body. Western medical structuralists carelessly destroyed immune organs, whereas Eastern functionalists developed practical methods to improve their operation. Research on the effects of the Chinese medicinal mushrooms in animals and humans shows them to stimulate immune function. For example, *Ganoderma* increases immune destruction of tumor cells and virus-infected cells, effects that are especially desirable in view of Western medicine's relative inability to treat cancer and viral infections successfully.

When I look at the body from a functional perspective, I see that defense is actually one component of a superfunction that I call *healing*. In *Spontaneous Healing* I tried to convey a sense of the manifold operations of the healing system, pointing out, for example, that even at the most fundamental level of life, the DNA molecule that encodes genetic information and directs all cellular processes, it is possible to observe an inherent ability to recognize injury or malfunction, to remove damaged structure, and to regenerate intact structure. If a strand of DNA is damaged—say, by an energetic ultraviolet ray from the sun—the molecule identifies the point of injury and repairs it, by manufacturing specific repair enzymes to do the job. The healing system operates from that fundamental level up to the level of cut fingers and into the mental realm, where it helps us adjust to emotional shocks. It operates continually, keeping most of us in good health most of the time in spite of all the agents of illness and forces of disorder that surround us constantly, and it is always at the ready to help us deal with serious threats to health when they arise.

To illustrate the potential for healing—a subject that conventional medical teaching, research, and practice largely ignore, by the way—I presented a number of cases in *Spontaneous Healing* from my experience with people who underwent dramatic reversals of life-threatening diseases like aplastic anemia and metastatic kidney cancer as well as more commonplace conditions like arthritis and back pain. Since the publication of that book, I have gathered many more healing stories, some from people who roused their healing systems to action by following the kinds of advice presented in the Eight-Week Program that is the subject of this book. I will recount some of those tales here to help motivate you to undertake the program and follow it through to its conclusion: a new and improved lifestyle that will increase your chances of enjoying optimum health into old age.

I also continue to scan the medical literature for evidence that my profession is beginning to take an interest in this type of healing. For now I see just the merest beginnings of movement, but I did come across a remarkable report in the July 1996 issue of the journal *Nature Genetics* that I want to share with you.

According to a team of researchers at the New York University Medical School, Jordan Houghton, a young boy from Michigan with an inherited fatal disease of the immune system, who should have been dead by age four, is now alive and in excellent health at age thirteen, not because of medical treatment but because his body somehow repaired the faulty genes he got from both parents. The disease, known as ADA deficiency, is a rare condition, occurring in about one in a million births; it killed the patient's brother at eighteen months. The defective genes fail to produce a functioning version of ADA, a vital enzyme needed to eliminate substances that can poison immune cells. Lacking that natural defense, the immune system is crippled, leaving ADA-deficient children susceptible to overwhelming infections from infancy. Medical doctors attempt to treat them by administering injections of the missing enzyme or by performing bone-marrow transplants, as well as by using aggressive antibiotic therapy to contain the infections.

Like his brother (who died four years before he was born), Jordan had many infections in infancy and grew slowly. Examination of his blood cells clearly showed that he had inherited defective copies of the key gene from both his mother and father. But by age two, Jordan began responding well to conventional medication, whereas his brother had not. He never needed enzyme injections or a bone-marrow transplant, and around age five, he suddenly started doing very well. Today he is a very active teenager and an A student who hardly ever gets colds. Some of his blood cells still show the faulty genes, but in some only the copy inherited from his father is flawed and the maternal gene is normal. Jordan's healing system managed to make a precise repair in the maternal gene, perhaps in just one blood cell initially. That cell was then able to multiply until Jordan's body could produce enough of the normal enzyme to permit his immune system to function correctly.

Talk about spontaneous healing! Of course, events like this are extremely rare, but I insist on taking them into account in trying to develop a picture of the full potential of the human healing system. When I look at common ailments—headaches, allergies, sinus conditions, digestive disorders, back pain, anxiety—I find healing to be the rule rather than the exception. Most illnesses are self-limited. They come to an end—just as a cut finger heals—because the healing system is able to handle most problems and restore the balance of health.

When illness persists, the healing system is blocked, stalled, or overwhelmed and needs help. The true purpose of medicine is to facilitate healing; the aim of treatment should be to unblock the healing system and allow it to do its work. Please keep in mind the distinction between healing and treatment: treatment originates from outside, whereas healing comes from within. Let me quote from *Spontaneous Healing:*

Suppose I come down with bacterial pneumonia, a serious, possibly life-threatening infection of the lungs. I go to a hospital, receive intravenous antibiotics, recover, and am discharged, cured. What caused the cure? Most people, doctors and patients alike, would say it was the treatment. But I want you to consider a different interpretation. Antibiotics reduce the numbers of invading germs to a point where the immune system can take over and finish the job. The real cause of the cure is the immune system, which may be unable to end an infection because it is overwhelmed by sheer numbers of bacteria and whatever toxic products they might make. Of course, the immune system is itself a component of the healing system.

I maintain that the final common cause of all cures is the healing system, whether or not treatment is applied. When treatments work, they do so by activating innate healing mechanisms. Treatment—including drugs and surgery—can facilitate healing and remove obstacles to it, but treatment is not the same as healing.

The best treatment is the least—the least invasive, least drastic, least expensive—that activates spontaneous healing.

And prevention always supersedes treatment in importance. Whether the focus of prevention is external, as in disinfecting drinking water, or internal, as in taking antioxidant supplements and natural tonics that boost immunity, preventing disease is always easier, cheaper, and surer than treating disease, so important that you must learn how to do it. You may go on the Eight-Week Program for any of a number of good reasons—to feel better, to get more energy, to lose weight, for instance—but its ultimate purpose is to reduce your risks of premature illness and death by enhancing the performance of your body's healing system.

A friend who is just turning forty lamented to me recently that he was getting to the age when bodies break down. "I think the human body comes with a forty-year warranty," he told me, "and after that it starts to go to hell." I replied that I thought the body was designed for considerably longer service, but he countered that in his world large numbers of his contemporaries were dropping. "Every time the phone rings, I hear about someone else just diagnosed with cancer," he went on. "Or, if it's not cancer, it's something else you don't want to have."

There is no doubt that many men and women have their first serious brush with disastrous loss of health in middle age, but I believe many of the disasters could be averted, because they are diseases of lifestyle, products of years of failing to eat wisely, exercise appropriately, or treat body and mind in ways that protect the healing system. In one sense, it is too bad that younger bodies are so forgiving. People in their teens, twenties, and early thirties can get away with eating quantities of fast food, with using stimulants and depressants, carousing, and abusing their bodies in all the ways our society seems to encourage. What I think happens around age forty, however, is not that the warranty runs out but that the bill comes due. That is, the cumulative effects of unhealthy habits and patterns of living make themselves known for the first time, as the natural resilience of the body inevitably begins to diminish. If young people could immediately feel the consequences of their lifestyles, I am sure most of them would clean up their acts early on. As it is, many see no reason to change, and some are shocked to discover that their bodies can "suddenly" fail in middle age. Actually, I think most bodies come with warranties for eighty years of productive, relatively trouble-free service, if basic requirements for preventive maintenance are followed. I have incorporated those requirements into the Eight-Week Program. If you complete it and make the core concepts part of your ongoing lifestyle, you will greatly reduce your risk of falling into the common traps that kill and disable people prematurely, leading to heart disease or cancer contracted in what should be the prime of life.

Nonetheless, it is certain that every one of us, sooner or later, will face a health crisis, and many of us will have to deal with doctors, hospitals, and all the contrivances of modern medicine. The question is not *if* such a crisis will occur but *when.* By making the Eight-Week Program part of your life, you can increase the likelihood that the when will be later rather than sooner. Still, I want to tell you why I think it is important to anticipate health crises and prepare for them.

Earlier this year, an acquaintance of mine, a writer in his early forties, finally decided to do something about the digestive symptoms he had ignored for almost two years. He had had persistent heartburn, stomach upsets, reflux, and intolerances to foods and drinks that he used to be able to enjoy. Despite the urgings of family and friends, he refused to see a doctor, lived on antacids, and tried to wish his symptoms away. Only when he could no longer swallow without difficulty did he visit a physician, and the news he got quickly turned from bad to worse. Endoscopic examination revealed a tumor mass near the lower end of his esophagus; a biopsy confirmed the suspicion that it was esophageal cancer, and he was scheduled for immediate surgery to remove the tumor and check for spread. Esophageal cancer is one of the hardest forms of cancer to treat; very few people who have it are alive five years after diagnosis.

Now I watched an unhappy and familiar scene unfold. The patient, who was of course terrified, found himself at the center of a drama in which family, friends, and health professionals came at him with their own agendas and their own ideas as to what was best for him. His younger sister, a yoga instructor and vegetarian, put him on a raw-foods diet and tried to get him to go with her to an alternative-cancer-treatment center in Mexico. His wife, the daughter of a cardiologist, forbade him to do so, and implored him to place his trust in the oncologists at the prestigious medical institution in New York where he was to undergo surgery. His friends inundated him with inspirational books about healing. One gave him a tome on Taoist philosophy with the admonition that he must read it before his surgery. Another friend downloaded information from the Internet about alternative treatments for esophageal cancer. I told the patient to try to find a hypnotherapist who could prepare him for the operation, particularly to make an audiotape with healing suggestions that he could listen to in the operating room, while under anesthesia. But surgery was just two days away; how could he find a hypnotherapist in time?

I describe this scene as unhappy because it is impossible to make careful decisions about life-and-death matters in the midst of such turmoil, with so many people pulling on you in different directions. This man was going to have to decide quickly whether to take the conventional treatments that would be pressed on him by oncologists after his surgery or whether to entrust himself to alternative therapies. He needed good advice about how to live with the diagnosis of cancer, how to eat, how to use his mind to help his healing system, but where was he going to get this practical information? Probably not in a volume of Taoist philosophy. Not only was he adrift with his own fear and ignorance, he was losing his autonomy with every step he took toward the operating room, and growing more confused by the day as he listened to all the conflicting stories from relatives, friends, and doctors.

I describe this scene as familiar because I have seen it too many times. Most people find themselves completely unprepared for major health crises and wind up scrambling desperately to maintain autonomy and develop sensible plans of action. Please try to prevent this from happening to you by thinking through in advance—now, while you are in good health—how you want to be treated when your health is in the balance, and whom you want to be in your inner circle of advisers. It is not too soon to be looking for a physician who knows conventional medicine and is open to using alternative treatments, for a skilled guided-imagery therapist or hypnotherapist, for a practitioner of traditional Chinese medicine, or for other people you would like to have on your support team. Nor is it too early to begin learning techniques that will help you maintain equanimity through trying circumstances, such as breath control, meditation, and cultivation of calmness and acceptance of change.

The Eight-Week Program includes aspects that will help you in this direction. I have designed it to be preventive in a very broad sense. It gives you the information you need to keep your healing system in optimal working order so that you can stay healthy as you encounter the obstacles and challenges of day-to-day life. It shows you how to build a lifestyle that will protect you from premature disability and death. It teaches practices and skills that will enable you to prepare body, mind, and spirit for any eventual health crises you may face. Start it now and reap the benefits for the rest of your life.

A HEALING STORY:
DEFYING A PROGNOSIS

HEATHER THOMPSON of Eugene, Oregon, sent me this account:

In 1984, when I was twenty-three years old, after being told by several gynecologists that I merely had PMS, I was finally diagnosed with a grapefruit-sized endometrial tumor that had ripped my uterus and ovaries from their "moorings," leaving them in the bottom of my abdominal cavity. I required surgery and then used Depo-Provera [an injectable, synthetic form of progesterone] for one year at the insistence of my surgeon. After that year, feeling "freaked out" and with a sense that tumors were growing again, I quit taking the pharmaceuticals and went to a nutritionist who diagnosed me with a severe candida [yeast] infection. I changed my diet accordingly, began to take chlorella [an algae supplement] to clean out the pharmaceutical build-up, and began to answer the question, "If I didn't have this disease at birth, what started it?" Hormones in milk and meat, I suspect, and being treated with repeated doses of antibiotics as a teenager, among other things. I now consume only the purest food, water, and air, and I've been in perfect health for ten years now, better than any time since I was a preteen. When stresses get too much, and it feels as though adhesions may be present, I go to my acupuncturist, and afterward I notice a marked improvement.

The prognosis given to me by my surgeon was: "You will have several more surgeries in the next five to ten years. You will be in pain a great deal. You will probably never conceive, and you definitely won't be able to sustain a pregnancy; giving birth would be a miracle. We just left your ovaries and uterus in case we discover a cure for endometriosis."

Well, it's amazing what natural remedies can do. Twelve years after the surgery, with a clean diet and a little assistance from Mother Nature, including herbal remedies from raspberry and nettles, my body is now ready to conceive and carry a baby to term.

3

THE WHOLE PICTURE

HUMAN BEINGS ARE BODIES, minds, and spirits. Health necessarily involves all of those components, and any program intended to improve health must address all of them. Conventional medicine pays almost exclusive attention to our physical bodies, giving lip service to our minds but not really taking them seriously, and totally ignoring our spirits. In spite of a great deal of research demonstrating the causative role of stress in illness and the interplay of emotions and immunity, most medical researchers and practitioners assume that physical causes can explain all diseases and that physical treatments—drugs, usually—are the only ones that count. I include under the heading "mind" our thoughts, beliefs, fantasies, and emotions; if medicine neglects the importance of these factors as influences on health, it hasn't a clue about the relevance of spiritual ones.

For an illustration of how far medicine in this century has moved toward a materialistic and mechanistic view of human beings, I need only point to the field of psychiatry, once a noble enterprise—the word "psychiatry" comes from Greek roots meaning "soul doctoring"—now reduced to a branch of pharmaceutical science. The field is dominated completely by a biomedical model that views all disturbed mentation as a result of disturbed brain chemistry and so offers us drugs as the only treatments worth using.

Many people consider spirit to be in the province of religion, but I insist on making a clear distinction between spirituality and religion. Spirituality has to do with the nonphysical, immaterial aspects of our beings—with energies, essences, and the part of us that existed before and will exist after the disintegration of the body. Religion attempts to institutionalize spirituality, and much of what goes on in its name concerns perpetuation of the institutions more than the welfare of individuals. It is possible to lead a spiritual life and explore the influence of spirituality on health whether you are religious or not. In the Eight-Week Program I will prescribe activities designed to raise spiritual energy with the aim of optimizing overall health; these activities have no religious connotations, and I hope no one will find them in conflict with any religious beliefs.

One of the disappointments of my professional life is meeting so few teachers who see the whole picture of health, who understand the importance of working on all fronts: the physical, the mental, and the spiritual. A few weeks ago, for example, I had dinner with a doctor who runs an established and respected residential program for improving health and longevity based on a very low-fat diet and regular exercise. He looked healthy and fit and had great confidence that his program could prevent and reverse many serious forms of illness, especially cardiovascular disease. The day before, news reports of an article in *JAMA* (*Journal of the American Medical Association*) had caught my eye. Researchers presented evidence that emotional risk factors for heart attacks might be more important than physical ones—that anger and deprivation of love might overshadow the contribution of serum cholesterol to the likelihood of a coronary. When I mentioned the reports, my dinner companion, who had not heard the news, scoffed. "What a bunch of baloney!" he said. Why was I not surprised by his reaction? I knew that his program paid little attention to the minds of patients and suspected that the news would threaten his world-view. He had part of the picture of health in very clear focus but chose not to expand his vision.

Here is a different example. I received in the mail a set of audiotapes recorded by a health writer and philosopher who teaches that all illness is emotional—that chronic back pain is the bodily expression of lack of emotional support, breast cancer the result of bottled-up anger, and AIDS the manifestation of guilt about unhealthy sexuality. I listened to the tapes, as much as I could stand of them, and discovered that the only strategy they offered to sick people was emotional-process work to release repressed feelings: ignore the physical body, they preached, and work only with the mind.

Some years ago, I did an intensive meditation retreat that involved long hours of sitting meditation interspersed with some walking meditation. One of the difficulties for me was not having an opportunity to exercise, since I had long enjoyed daily aerobic activity. When I had an interview with the spiritual teacher who led the retreat, I told him of my frustration. His reply was that exercise would be a diversion of attention away from meditation. "When you begin to experience the body as energy, the idea of physical exercise seems gross," he went on. "You can accomplish the same thing just by circulating energy." I disagree.

In recent years, as I was doing research for this book and the Eight-Week Program, I visited a number of spas that offer training in fitness and healthy living. Again, I found only parts of the picture of health, not the whole. Many programs placed lopsided emphasis on the physical body, ignoring mind and spirit. Some served low-fat dishes with few or no animal products but had no awareness of the importance of organic foods. One that had its dietary act together discouraged clients from using supplements. Several served chlorinated water. At one spa that served vegan cuisine (no animal food), whose medical director condemned eggs, cheese, and fish as "poisons," maintenance men sprayed the grounds with chemical pesticides and herbicides daily; it was impossible to walk around without inhaling some of the fumes.

The program in this book works with the whole picture of health. I will ask you to examine and make changes in all the components of lifestyle that contribute to health, not just to improve your diet and increase your exercise. I will teach you breathing techniques that help neutralize stress and smooth out emotional swings. I will recommend the use of vitamins, minerals, and herbs that I have found to boost the body's healing system. I will give you advice about protecting yourself from toxins in food, water, and air. And I will suggest practices—such as bringing more beauty into your life—that are good for your spirit.

This is the same way that I work with patients. Because illness is always multifactorial, I always ask those with medical problems to work on many different fronts at once. Look at the problem of coronary heart disease, a leading killer in our culture, one that many of us need to be concerned about so that we can take protective measures. Heart attacks kill and disable many middle-aged men and many postmenopausal women, and it is clear that many of the deaths are preventable, since coronary heart disease is essentially a disease of lifestyle, rare or nonexistent in some societies in which people live very differently from the way we do. One large and influential school of medical thought sees elevated serum cholesterol as the main risk factor for heart attack and focuses all of its efforts in this direction— by urging people to eat low-fat diets, especially avoiding food sources of cholesterol and saturated fat, and by prescribing many doses of cholesterol-lowering drugs. Of course exercise is recommended, too, since it is good for everything, cardiovascular health included.

Yet there are splinter groups of physicians and researchers who question the centrality of cholesterol in the genesis of heart attacks. One theory that I am willing to consider sees atherosclerosis as an imbalance in a natural healing process. In this view, the primary defect in coronary heart disease is weakness of the intima (the lining of the arteries); the body attempts to repair cracks in the intima by plugging them with cholesterol, a natural and necessary substance. Coronary arteries, being subjected to regular, incessant, mechanical stress from the contraction of the heart, are more likely to develop cracks if their linings are weak. And what might cause weakness of the intima? One strong possibility is vitamin-C deficiency, since that vitamin is necessary for the production of strong connective tissue. The only animals subject to coronary heart disease other than primates are guinea pigs and pigs, which, like us, have lost the ability to synthesize vitamin C and must get it from dietary sources. Since vitamin C is harmless, why not take enough of it to make sure our bodies can make strong lining tissue for our arteries?

Another line of research looks to the clotting tendency of the blood as a risk factor equal to or greater than elevated serum cholesterol. Even if the coronary arteries are narrowed by atherosclerotic plaque, heart attacks cannot occur unless blood clots form in them. We know many ways to "thin" the blood: aspirin, garlic, vitamin E, fish oils, and alcohol all do it, and it is likely that psychological factors play a role as well, since stress may affect the clotting system. So why not recommend natural blood-thinners in appropriate amounts, and stress-reduction training, along with advice about lowering serum cholesterol?

And that's not all. Even if blood supply to the heart muscle is temporarily interrupted, the consequences are not predictable. Some people drop dead, others recover and go on to become healthier and more active than they were before. What makes the difference? More than the location and extent of the injury, the determining factor may be the state of the heart and body in general. In particular, if the sympathetic (arousing) branch of the involuntary nervous system dominates at the time of the attack, the heart muscle might be predisposed to go into ventricular fibrillation, the chaotic, useless movement that leads to death within minutes. On the other hand, if the parasympathetic (relaxing) nerves are dominant, the heart muscle may be protected from this catastrophe even though the area of injury is extensive. Sympathetic dominance correlates with chronic anxiety, stress, and a tendency to rage when frustrated. Parasympathetic dominance correlates with openness, calm, and acceptance. It seems to me we should all take note of these facts whatever our serum cholesterol levels are.

For very good reasons, most people associate emotions with the heart; some people even experience emotional disruptions as pain or discomfort in the chest. Our feelings interact with our hearts through complex nervous and hormonal systems of communication, which can also affect the condition of our coronary arteries. One type of coronary event that can precipitate a heart attack is a spasm of those vessels in response to an emotional upheaval. In the Eight-Week Program, I advise you, as a spiritual exercise, to try to heal damaged relationships—for instance, by extending forgiveness to someone who has hurt you. My experience is that the act of forgiving heals the forgiver, and along with many other components of the body, the coronary arteries might be beneficiaries of the healing energies released.

In other words, even if your particular goal is a limited one, such as avoiding a heart attack, you must attend to the whole picture just as much as anyone else. It is not enough to cut your intake of saturated fat. It is not enough to take cholesterol-lowering agents, whether natural or synthetic. It is not enough to increase your exercise. It is not enough to practice stress reduction. *To optimize the function of the healing system, you must do everything in your power to improve physical health, mental/emotional health, and spiritual health.*

A Healing Story:
The Spiritual Roots of Health

Diana Hydzik, a doctor in Chicago, sent me this story of her experience with a chronic and painful joint disease:

I was diagnosed in 1990 with seronegative arthropathy [noninfectious joint destruction] at age forty-one, during my fourth year of medical school. I had left an abusive marriage in 1987 and spent the first two years in medical school in court and depositions during a very contentious divorce. When it was finally all over, I became sick. I had a few abnormal blood tests, and X-rays showed cartilage destruction in my wrists. I finally sought the advice of a rheumatologist due to overwhelming fatigue, which threatened my capacity to finish medical school. I could not stay awake through the day, even if I slept twelve hours at night. Prednisone enabled me to finish school (six weeks late) as well as one year of residency. I felt the other usual drugs [for autoimmune arthritis] would be destructive to my general health, and therefore left residency and sought alternative methods of treatment. I began working in rural emergency departments, which gave me time to rest, read, and travel to consult alternative practitioners.

Initially, I consulted a chiropractor who trained in Europe. He recommended fish-oil supplements and herbal treatment for yeast infection of the bowel. I experienced considerable improvement, though no further improvement with his other treatments. I next consulted a Chinese doctor, who analyzed my pulses and tongue monthly and prescribed an herbal mixture which I boiled and drank three times a day—this designed to reduce "damp heat in my bowel." I also went for acupuncture, which was very effective initially but became less so over time. I tapered down the prednisone by one-milligram steps, while I began taking vitamins and DHEA [a hormone supplement, useful in autoimmunity]. I gave up coffee completely as an experiment, and my diet became nearly vegetarian. (I got carry-out from a health-food store.) I also eliminated dairy products.

As a former psychologist I was very open to exploring the mind-body connection. In fact, it was the reason I went to medical school, although I had no time to study it. I began practicing relaxation and visualization and got regular massage therapy. After the first eighteen months of alternative treatment, I was able to stop the prednisone completely, using some NSAIDs [nonsteroidal anti-inflammatory drugs] as needed.

However, in the summer of 1994, I again became worse, developing knee effusions and calf spasms. I stopped the Chinese herbs and returned to prednisone. I changed my diet further and pursued energy work (reiki and healing touch), which provided temporary relief. Most importantly, I became involved with transformational imagery, which gave me a means to access cellular memory. I also started taking two very beneficial supplements: shark cartilage and the herb boswellia.

The past year has brought almost complete resolution of my symptoms. I went to Sedona, Arizona, last year and had such dramatic experiences there, I felt it held the source for my healing. I gave up a full-time contract and have been working *locum tenens* [as a part-time substitute] to have time and flexibility to pursue my healing. I've been to Sedona sixteen weeks this year, primarily involved with a combination of breath work, imagery, Eastern spirituality, and energy medicine and environmental medicine. I had the amalgam fillings and a root canal removed from my mouth, had chelation therapy for any mercury in my system, and treatment for an intestinal parasite.

Most significant, however, has been coming to see my illness as a crisis of my spirit: of coming to terms with my life experiences, my purpose, and the source of all existence. While I had had spiritual experiences with different healers prior to this year, my resistance to spirituality caused me to dismiss them as coincidences, which I was willing to use for healing but did not consider "real." I thought faith healing was effective for believers, but I was, after all, a scientist. I now believe that the spiritual work has been what truly brought healing, while all the supplements and treatments only gave me symptomatic relief—until I could accomplish the spiritual growth I needed.

A Healing Story:
Better Breathing

In 1990, Rachel H., a lawyer from San Francisco, consulted me about her diagnosis of Parkinson's disease. She told me that, five years before, her left knee had begun to buckle under her on walks, and she had developed progressive stiffness of her left arm and leg. After visits to orthopedists and eventual knee surgery, she was thought to have multiple sclerosis, but finally the neurologists agreed that the problem was an unusual form of Parkinson's disease. Subsequently, she wrote about her experiences with conventional and alternative medicine for management of her illness. Recently she wrote me:

> I have continued the regimen of alternative/Eastern efforts I described in my recent article. They include acupuncture, yoga, massage, meditation, and other stress-reduction work.
>
> The biggest challenge since my diagnosis was the onset, in about 1990, of occasional (once every few weeks or so) seizures during sleep. I responded by searching for alternatives to seizure medication and eventually found respiratory biofeedback, which identified a pattern of "chronic hyperventilation" (shallow, too-frequent breathing). This appeared to be part of a long-standing syndrome, including an absence of lower-abdominal breathing, poor posture, constriction around the diaphragm area, cold hands and feet. I entirely changed this pattern (over time) by combining the biofeedback sessions with work with my yoga instructor, bodyworker, and

counselor. I changed posture and other things that were affecting my body structure and breathing and presumably skewing the oxygen/carbon-dioxide mix. As I began to change my breathing system, the seizures diminished in frequency and severity, finally—two years after the first one—stopping altogether. I have had none since May 1993.

4

WHY EIGHT WEEKS?

IN WORKING WITH PATIENTS, I commonly recommend lifestyle changes in addition to natural remedies. Recently, a woman in her early sixties consulted me about osteoarthritis, which restricted the use of her hands and caused considerable pain in many other joints as well. Her family physician prescribed several different NSAIDs, but she could not tolerate any of them. Because they upset her stomach and made her feel "spacy," she tried to use them only when the pain became intolerable and she could not get relief from hot baths, topical remedies, or other simple methods she had learned from friends and from books.

I wrote out a list of suggestions for her, all intended to reduce inflammation in her body. I began by explaining that dietary fats either promote or retard inflammation. In the former category are all polyunsaturated vegetable oils—corn, sesame, sunflower, safflower, and the like—margarine, and other artificially hydrogenated fats, including all partially hydrogenated vegetable oils and products made from them. I asked her to eliminate all of these from her diet. Instead she was to rely on olive oil and eat oily fish such as salmon, mackerel, sardines, and herring. These fish provide special fatty acids, the omega-3s, that retard inflammation. She was also to take a supplement of evening-primrose oil, source of another desirable fatty acid, called GLA. Her diet was not bad, but I urged her to eat still fewer animal foods, more whole-grain products, and more fresh vegetables. I also told her to take two common spices on a regular basis, ginger and turmeric, both of which are natural anti-inflammatory agents. I gave her a basic antioxidant formula of vitamins and minerals to take every day, one that you will learn to use when you follow the Eight-Week Program, and I suggested that she try to swim regularly, since swimming is the best form of exercise for anyone with sore joints. Finally, I referred her to an acupuncturist for symptomatic relief by a drugless method.

After following this regimen for a month, the patient reported slight improvement in her condition and consequent slight reduction in her use of the prescribed NSAIDs. About three weeks later, she experienced marked improvement and was able to dispense with the pharmaceuticals entirely. Since then, her arthritis has been contained, leaving her free of pain most of the time.

Why do NSAIDs give pain relief within hours, whereas the natural approach takes weeks? Actually, both methods work on the same physiological endpoint: a family of hormones called *prostaglandins* that mediate pain and inflammation. I should explain that inflammation, despite the discomfort it causes us, is a natural component of the body's healing response. It is the visible and perceptible aspect of immune activity intended to contain infection and injury and promote repair of damaged tissue. But too much of a good thing is never good, and when an inflammatory response becomes too intense or persists too long, inflammation itself produces disease rather than healing. Prostaglandins regulate this powerful response of the immune system. Like most of the body's regulatory substances, they occur as a family that divides into two functional branches—one that promotes inflammation and one that holds it in check. In health, these opposing biochemical forces are in balance, so that inflammation occurs only where and when it is needed for defense and repair, does not become too strong, and ends on schedule. Too much promotion and too much suppression of inflammation are both unbalanced states that lead to disease.

The anti-inflammatory drugs that have become so popular among doctors and patients in recent years antagonize the actions of those prostaglandins that promote inflammation. As with most pharmacological antagonists, their effect is rapid and often dramatic, but it comes at a price. There are side effects—toxicity—in this case, irritation of the lining of the stomach that can produce symptoms as mild as heartburn and as major as death from sudden gastric hemorrhage. Thousands of patients on NSAIDs die every year from the latter calamity. In addition, treatment with pharmacological antagonists often results in a rebound of symptoms as soon as treatment stops, so that patients become dependent on the drugs. As soon as they try to reduce the dose or stop taking the pills entirely, their inflammation and attendant pain and immobility return full-force. This pattern is quite logical. The body always strives for *homeostasis,* a word derived from Greek roots meaning "same place." That is, the body seeks equilibrium, so that, if it experiences an outside force, it pushes back against it in order to attempt to stay where it is. Anti-inflammatory drugs are strong forces from outside, and homeostasis requires that the body mount a counteractive effort to balance them, in this case by producing more of the promoting prostaglandins. Whenever patients try to stop using the drugs, they experience an increase in symptoms because their overabundance of those hormones is now unopposed.

The natural approach aims for the same result—restoring balance in the prostaglandin system—but accomplishes its end in a different manner. The body makes prostaglandins out of fatty acids from dietary sources. Some fatty acids, like those in safflower oil, corn oil, and margarine, favor the synthesis of prostaglandins that promote inflammation; others, like the omega-3s in fish oils and GLA, favor synthesis of the inhibitory prostaglandins. Manipulation of the prostaglandin system through dietary adjustment works, but it takes time, producing a gradual shift in the balance of hormone production. The advantages that offset the delay are freedom from toxicity and avoidance of dependence on drugs. When you change hormonal balance gradually by changing diet, you do not disturb the body's homeostasis and do not have to contend with rebounding of symptoms.

There is another, subtler advantage of the natural approach that I should mention, since I am a firm believer in mind/body interactions and their potential to create both disease and health. It is obvious to me that the mind can dramatically influence inflammation, presumably through the medium of chemical messengers—neuropeptides—produced in the brain that interact directly with immune cells, either activating or suppressing them. I won't go into the details of this influence except to note that well-known studies of hypnosis demonstrate that inflammatory responses on the skin of subjects in trance can be induced or prevented by suggestion, and these effects are immediate. A hypnotist can touch a subject in deep trance with a finger, representing it as a piece of hot metal, and a blister will appear at the site of contact. Conversely, suggestion can prevent blistering in response to contact with a real piece of hot metal. Blistering is an aspect of the inflammatory mechanism, mediated by hormones that cause blood vessels in the skin to become leaky, allowing serum to flow between the outer and inner layers of the skin.

The placebo response—a therapeutic result produced by belief in a treatment—contributes to the efficacy of all drugs and may well play a significant role in successful outcomes with nonsteroidal anti-inflammatory agents, adding to their direct pharmacological actions. Certainly, the placebo response may play a role in any favorable outcome of a program of dietary adjustment and the use of mild, natural anti-inflammatory agents like ginger and turmeric. As a practitioner of mind/body medicine, I consider the placebo response my greatest ally. I view it as a pure healing response from within and want to encourage it as much as I can. I know that the dietary changes I suggested for the woman with osteoarthritis could shift her prostaglandin system in the right direction. I also know that it is very difficult for people to change their habits of eating, so that, if they are willing to do so, they are committing significant mental energy to healing. Placebo responses may appear very quickly when people take prescribed drugs, but they disappear as soon as the drugs are discontinued. When they develop in response to changes in lifestyle, they may appear slowly and build over time but then take root and become an ongoing contribution to health.

My experience is that responses to natural medicine occur more slowly than responses to suppressive drugs. Based on my observations of many patients who have used natural therapeutic agents and changes in lifestyle to control various ailments, I feel that a minimum of six to eight weeks is required for someone to notice the effects of such programs.

Here is another case to illustrate the point. A thirty-six-year-old man came to me complaining of indigestion and heartburn. The symptoms were so frequent that he was used to eating over-the-counter antacid tablets regularly. He was a lawyer in a stressful job, happily married, who drank four cups of coffee a day, had one alcoholic drink after work, played competitive racquetball for exercise, and ate reasonably healthy meals at home but often lunched out with clients and usually indulged in heavy Mexican food. Although the lawyer's recent physical examination, including blood studies, was normal, his doctor suggested a trial of a prescription drug to suppress acid production in the stomach. In listening to this man's answers to my many questions about his life, I came to feel that he was essentially healthy, with problems in the areas of diet, habits, and the handling of stress.

I gave him a program to follow, beginning with an elimination of coffee, a known stomach irritant. I suggested adjustments in his diet, including different kinds of restaurants to visit and foods to order when he ate out. I taught him a breathing exercise for relaxation, one that I will teach you in the Eight-Week Program. I told him I was not opposed to his use of alcohol but thought he might want to stop drinking until his stomach symptoms resolved, especially if he could use breathing and exercise as a way to unwind from his daily routine. I explored with him the possibility of building up an exercise routine that was not based on a competitive sport and discovered that he used to be an avid cyclist but now used his bicycle only rarely. Finally, I told him about a licorice extract (called DGL) that he could get at any health food store to replace the antacids and prescribed drug. (Licorice builds up the mucous coating of the stomach lining, making it more resistant to the irritating effect of acid.) Because this patient did not want to get involved with more medical tests and pharmaceutical drugs and suspected that his symptoms were a call to make changes in his life, he accepted these recommendations and seemed to me willing to try to implement them. I asked him to call me at monthly intervals with reports on his progress.

When he first reported back, after one month, he told me that he had found some suggestions easy and others not so easy. Taking the licorice extract was easy and helped him wean himself away from antacids. Practicing the breathing exercise was easy and rewarding, because he could feel its relaxing effect immediately. Getting off coffee was hard. He cut down to two cups a day but could not do without those, because then he was too tired in the morning to face a workday. He was trying to alter his patterns of eating out, but his bicycle was still gathering dust in the garage. Instead of having his after-work drink every day, he was down to every other day. His stomach symptoms were "a little better." I told him he was doing well, to take it step by step, and to make a special effort to break his dependence on coffee. I suggested he try a grain-based coffee substitute or an herbal tea such as chamomile or peppermint, both of which soothe the stomach. If he found he simply could not get along without caffeine, I advised him to try Japanese green tea as a coffee replacement. Not only is green tea free of most of the stomach irritants in coffee, it also offers several health benefits that coffee does not. (It has cholesterol-lowering and cancer-preventive effects.)

The two-month follow-up was even better. He was drinking two cups of green tea in the morning instead of coffee, and although this was a difficult adjustment and he still missed his coffee, his stomach felt so much better that he was happy with the change. He was enthusiastic about the breathing exercise. "I think I'm addicted to it," he said, "but it's a healthy addiction." He had started to cycle after work, playing racquetball on weekends and enjoying it more. His dining-out patterns were much better. He said he was sleeping more soundly and generally had more energy.

After one more month, he told me that he thought he did not need to talk to me again. He now used the licorice extract only occasionally, had almost no stomach distress, and was even able to eat a Mexican meal for lunch once in a while. He liked "a drink now and then with friends" but no longer had to have alcohol to relax at the end of a day of work.

This patient's experience with trying to change old habits is typical. By definition, habits are repetitive behavior; as such they are easy and familiar, the ruts we fall into while moving through life. Changing habits is hard, especially at first, requiring determined effort and time to make the changes stick. It took this man about two months to change his habit of drinking coffee, even though coffee was bothering his stomach.

What about making major changes in habits of eating or exercise, such as moving away from meat or starting to walk every day? I've made these recommendations to many patients who have consulted me, and I've watched people at spas and fitness centers trying to take the first steps. Again, I think there are two requirements for success: motivation and determination to initiate the change, along with time to practice the new patterns and have them become fixed. And, again, I observe that two months is a minimum period for this process.

Here is one more case in point. A young man in his late twenties consulted me about anxiety. He said he had always been high-strung and nervous; he had experienced symptoms like butterflies in his stomach and sweaty palms before exams in schools, sometimes with episodes of diarrhea. In the past few years, he had been subject to attacks of severe anxiety that began without warning, often when he was sitting at his desk. (He worked as a computer programmer at a university medical center.) He would begin to breathe rapidly and shallowly, feeling that he could not catch his breath. At the same time he would turn pale, and his skin would become cold and clammy. There was always a sense of apprehension, as if some catastrophe were about to befall him. These episodes lasted from a few minutes to over an hour and left him feeling exhausted and unable to concentrate for the rest of the day. A psychologist he had seen a few times had diagnosed him with anxiety disorder and had sent him to a doctor who prescribed an antianxiety drug, but the patient did not like the way it made him feel (it interfered with his alertness and memory at work). He was worried because the attacks were becoming more frequent.

This patient needed lifestyle medicine. His diet was passable; he used no alcohol, tobacco, caffeine, or other drugs; but he did not exercise, had no training in relaxation skills, was somewhat isolated socially, and spent—in my opinion—excessive time surfing the Internet and paying attention to world news, which generally upset him. I recommended daily walks and breath work, since I consider this to be a specific treatment for anxiety. I urged him to take news fasts, as I will urge you to do in the Eight-Week Program; lectured him about the dangers of Internet addiction; and sent him to a counselor who I thought might be able to help him work through his problem of social isolation. I also told him how to use tincture of passionflower, an herbal remedy sold in health-food stores, made from a native American plant (*Passiflora incarnata*) with very mild relaxant effects. The anxiety attacks had scared him enough to make him very compliant. He took all these suggestions readily and promised to follow through on them.

So he did. But after a month, he was disappointed not to see great progress and was strongly tempted to resume his old ways—to give up the walks and go back to the Internet and the news. The anxiety attacks were just as frequent. I simply told him to continue and be patient, particularly to practice the breathing exercise religiously, at least twice a day and whenever he felt the beginnings of anxiety. After another month, he reported that the attacks were decreasing in both frequency and severity, which motivated him to stick with the program, although he dispensed with the passionflower tincture because "I don't think it does anything for me." He felt "more energized and more confident" and said he could not now imagine a day without doing his breathing and walking. It was a full six months before the anxiety attacks stopped completely. By then, his new habits were part of his life, and he found that he could tolerate more time on the Internet and a little news without being thrown off balance. From my point of view, he turned the corner at two months, when his new, healthier patterns were just becoming habits.

Therefore, both from observing the effects of natural therapies and from watching people try to make lasting changes in how they live, I have concluded that two months—eight weeks—is the critical time, to see effects of therapeutic regimens as well as to replace old habits with new. Not that some changes may not appear much sooner or that more time may not be needed for others. But if you can follow a program of healthy living for two months, you will have made the commitment of time and energy necessary for it to work. If you follow the Eight-Week Program in this book to its conclusion, you will have begun to enhance the functioning of your body's healing system and to have set yourself on a lifelong course of optimum health.

And I hope that all of you who undertake it will have the kind of success these people did:

• Laura Tabaracci of Poughkeepsie, New York: "I have done Dr. Weil's Eight-Week Program! I have had wonderful results. My immune system seems to be stronger. I have learned to breathe differently and have an increased awareness of the way my body responds to different situations. I have been inspired to take a look at the way I was living."

• Dennis Stitz of Denville, New Jersey: "I followed your Eight-Week Program almost entirely (98 percent). I feel healthier physically, mentally, spiritually. I have more energy, I sleep better and fewer hours. I feel happier, calmer, less anxious. My immune system has become stronger. I don't catch colds. I don't get tired after an active day. My blood tests have improved. And I function better overall during the day."

PART TWO

THE EIGHT-WEEK PROGRAM

5

WEEK ONE

CONGRATULATIONS! You are about to embark on an exciting and healthy adventure of restyling your life in order to attain optimum health. I will give you specific directions for projects to do, as well as for changes to make in your diet and patterns of exercise. I will tell you about dietary supplements that are safe and effective, and I will also give you suggestions for taking advantage of the mind/body connection and for increasing spiritual energy. First I will outline the steps of this beginning week of the Eight-Week Program; then I will present an extensive commentary on each of the steps, so that you will understand the reasons for doing them. Let's begin!

Projects

• Start by going through your pantry and refrigerator to identify and discard common unhealthy foods. Throw out all oils other than olive oil and throw out any olive oil that smells old or rancid. Get rid of any margarine, solid vegetable shortenings, and products (such as cookies and crackers) made with them. Also discard any products made with cottonseed oil. Read the labels of all food products so that you can dispose of any containing partially hydrogenated oils of any kind. If you do not have any extra-virgin olive oil on hand, buy a bottle and start using it. You might also want to buy a small bottle of organic, expeller-pressed canola oil from the health-food store and some dark-roasted sesame oil from a Chinese or Japanese grocery store or the Asian-food section of the supermarket.

• Throw out any artificial sweeteners containing saccharin or aspartame and any products made with them.
• Throw out any products containing artificial coloring (indicated on the label by phrases like "color added," "artificially colored," or the name of a particular dye, such as "FD&C red #3").
• Make a commitment to read labels of all food products you buy. Pay special attention to the fat content, especially the saturated-fat content. I would like you to keep your total fat intake to about 20–25 percent of calories, and saturated-fat intake as low as possible. Do not buy products whose labels list more chemicals than recognizable ingredients.

Diet

• Start eating some fresh broccoli this week. If you like this vegetable and have favorite ways of preparing it, you know what to do. Otherwise, try the recipe on page 53. Have broccoli twice this week.
• Eat salmon, sardines, or kippers at least once this week. (You will find some great, easy salmon recipes beginning on page 54.) If you do not want to eat fish, buy some flaxseeds at a health-food store, grind them (directions are on page 52), and sprinkle them over your food once or twice this week.

Supplements

• Start taking vitamin C if you do not do so already: 1,000 to 2,000 milligrams with breakfast, another dose with dinner, and a third dose at bedtime, if convenient.

Exercise

• Try to walk ten minutes a day five days this week. If you are already on a program of aerobic exercise other than walking, do the walks in addition.

Mental/Spiritual

• Think about your own experiences of healing. Make a list of illnesses or injuries or problems you have recovered from in the past two years. Note down anything you did to speed the healing process.

• Begin to practice Breath Observation (see page 60) for five minutes every day.
• Buy some flowers to keep in your home, where you can enjoy them.

COMMENTARY

Projects

I've asked you to clear out your pantry and refrigerator of unhealthy foods, beginning with fats and oils. Here is the rationale for doing so:

Stale fats are extremely unhealthy. On exposure to air, fats oxidize. Polyunsaturated fats oxidize more readily than monounsaturated ones, and monounsaturated fats oxidize faster than saturated ones. Rates of oxidation increase with exposure to light and warmer temperatures. As oxidation progresses, fats become rancid, a condition easily detected by the human nose. Oxidized fats can damage DNA, promote the development of cancer, and speed up aging and degenerative changes in our tissues. Always smell oils before you use them, discarding any if you can detect even a hint of rancidity. It is also a good idea to get in the habit of smelling foods that contain fat before you eat them, especially nuts, chips, and snack foods, to make sure the oils have not oxidized. When you purchase oils, buy smaller rather than larger containers, keep them in the refrigerator, and use them up quickly.

The tendency to oxidize readily is the problem with most vegetable oils, particularly the polyunsaturated ones that fill the shelves of supermarkets: safflower, sunflower, corn, sesame, and soy. I recommend against using any of them. The only exception I make is for the dark-roasted sesame oil that is a popular ingredient in Chinese and Japanese cuisines. Its flavor is so intense that it can be used in small amounts—from a few drops to a teaspoon or two at most—to season soups and stir-fries at the end of cooking; it can also be used to make a great low-fat salad dressing (see recipe on page 56).

The best all-around oil to use is olive. Olive oil contains mostly monounsaturated fat, which seems much better for our bodies than either polyunsaturated or saturated fat. We seem to be able to process oleic acid, the principal fatty acid in olive oil, better than any other fatty acid, and populations that rely on olive oil as their main dietary fat have lower rates of both heart disease and cancer than

Americans and most Europeans do, even though their total fat intake is not that much lower. Remember that olive oil is still fat; eating it immoderately can raise cholesterol and contribute to obesity. In moderation it is a healthy ingredient that can make food much more appealing. Buy a good brand of extra-virgin olive oil—the result of the first, gentle pressing of the olives—so that you can enjoy its rich flavor. Let your eye and nose guide you: the best olive oils are green or greenish yellow and have a delightful fruity aroma. Professional cooks often discourage you from cooking with the extra-virgin form, because they say it should be reserved for salads and special dishes. I disagree. As with all oils, keep this one in the refrigerator to protect it from light, heat, and resultant oxidation. Olive oil will slowly so-lidify in the cold, but can easily be made pourable again by setting the bottle in hot water for a few minutes. (If you use it frequently, you can keep a small amount at room temperature for convenience.)

If you need to use oil in a dish you are preparing where the flavor of olive oil would be inappropriate, I suggest that you use canola oil, a neutral-flavored monounsaturated oil obtained from the seed of a plant related to mustard. In recent years, canola has acquired a repu-tation as a heart-healthy oil, but I consider it a distant runner-up to olive. Canola oil is not made up mostly of oleic acid, nor do we have epidemiological evidence, comparable to that for olive oil, of its asso-ciation with good health in populations that use a lot of it. In any case, the canola oil you will find in most grocery stores is not accept-able. It has been extracted with chemical solvents or by high-speed presses that generate high heat; both extraction methods alter fatty-acid chemistry in undesirable ways. (I'll explain more about this when I tell you why you have to throw out any margarine you might have on hand.) Furthermore, canola producers use a lot of pesticides on the crop, residues of which probably find their way into the final product. For these reasons, I recommend only organic, expeller-pressed canola oil, which you are most likely to find in natural-food stores.

On to margarine. It has two strikes against it that render it unfit for consumption by anyone wanting to attain optimum health. First, the process of hardening vegetable oils to create solid spreads in-creases the percentage of saturated fat and thereby diminishes any advantage over butter in the realm of cardiovascular friendliness. Second, and of even greater concern to me because it is a danger less recognized by doctors, the process of artificially hydrogenating oils deforms fatty acids, creating unnatural species called *trans*-fatty acids, or TFAs. Putting TFAs into your body may unbalance the hormonal systems that regulate healing, lead to the construction of defective cell membranes, and encourage the development of cancer.

If it comes to a choice between butter and margarine, always take butter. But I hope you will be able to reduce your butter consumption as well, because it is one of the highest sources of saturated fat in our diets, clearly implicated in atherosclerosis and arterial disease. It is possible to learn to enjoy really good bread with nothing on it, and to enjoy vegetables without butter or margarine. If you must put fat on bread, try a little olive oil or some mashed, seasoned avocado (a source of monounsaturated oil). You can also find in the refrigerators of natural-food stores new emulsified vegetable-oil spreads made without heat or hydrogenation.

For the same reasons that I reject margarine as a food, I also urge you to avoid all other sources of artificially hardened fats. Solid vegetable shortening is easy to do without. Much harder are all of the commercial products made with partially hydrogenated oils. Manufacturers like these unnatural fats because they oxidize less quickly than liquid oil, yielding longer shelf life. No matter how good are the oils that go into the process of partial hydrogenation, what comes out is unnatural and unhealthy, since it is full of TFAs. I predict that accumulating medical evidence about the harmfulness of partially hydrogenated oils will eventually force them out of food products. In the meantime, I cannot urge you too strongly to read labels carefully and reject all products containing them. Partially hydrogenated oils are ubiquitous in snack foods, baked goods, cookies, crackers, spreads, and many other items in grocery stores and supermarkets.

I've asked you to avoid cottonseed oil and anything made with it because it has too high a percentage of saturated fat, may contain natural toxins, and probably has unacceptably high levels of pesticide residues, since cotton is not classified as a food crop, and farmers use many agrichemicals when growing it. Again, get in the habit of reading labels carefully when you shop for food.

Fats are one of the three "macronutrients" we eat, the others being proteins and carbohydrates. There is now a great deal of information about how the amount and kind of fat we eat affects our health, and I will continue to summarize it for you in the commentaries that follow the week-by-week instructions. I will also give you

the most up-to-date facts I have about choosing proteins and carbohydrates wisely in order to protect and enhance your capacity for
natural healing.

The other products I asked you to throw away this first week are
foods containing artificial sweeteners, artificial colors, and large
numbers of chemical additives. These substances do not require
lengthy comment.

There is not a shred of evidence that the availability of artificial,
noncaloric sweeteners has helped anyone lose weight—the main reason for their popularity—and enough evidence of potential harm to
exclude them from a healthy diet. Saccharin, cyclamates, and aspartame (NutraSweet) all taste funny, and disturb physiology in some
people (causing headaches and menstrual dysfunction, for example).
Some experts suspect them of promoting cancer and having toxic effects on the nervous system. You are much better off eating moderate
amounts of sugar than any of these unnatural compounds.

Similarly, the chemicals used to dye foods, drugs, and cosmetics
are a suspect group of highly reactive molecules that may interact
with DNA in ways that increase mutation and malignant transformation of cells. Read labels and avoid them. I do not object to natural coloring agents like annatto (yellow/orange), beet (red/purple),
carotene (yellow/orange), chlorella (green), and caramel (brown).

Diet

The dietary changes recommended in the Eight-Week Program are
intended to move you in the direction of eating less fat (especially less
saturated fat), less animal protein, more whole grains and other complex carbohydrates, and more fruits and vegetables. This week I have
asked you to eat some fresh broccoli, one of the most healthful members of the cabbage family or crucifers. (The name means "cross-
bearer," referring to the pattern formed by the flower petals of plants
in this group.) Cruciferous vegetables have significant anticancer
properties; broccoli is most effective in this regard, and one of its
most important constituents, sulphoraphane, is even sold in tablet
form ("broccoli in a pill") in health-food stores. Of course, isolated
sulphoraphane is no more broccoli in a pill than beta-carotene is a
carrot. Broccoli has many nutrients and protective compounds in it,

as well as fiber. It also tastes good and is a source of pleasure in the diet if it is well prepared.

I have in my life encountered plenty of poorly prepared broccoli, which is anything but a source of pleasure. The easiest way to ruin this vegetable is to overcook it, turning it into a yellowish-green, malodorous mush. I am sure that most people who think they do not like broccoli know it only in that form. I do not recommend eating broccoli raw, because it does not taste especially good that way and may be less digestible. Perfectly cooked broccoli should be beautifully bright green and tender-crisp; my family and I like it really crunchy. That might require only five minutes of cooking or less, meaning you cannot put the pot on the stove and ignore it. Broccoli stalks are delicious if they are peeled properly, and a simple technique—peeling to beneath the fibrous layer—also renders the smaller stems more tender. It is true that the preparation of fresh vegetables takes time—not very much, in the case of broccoli—but what it really takes is knowledge of how to maximize flavor, appearance, and nutritive value. I hope you will begin to experiment with new vegetables and ways of preparing them. Scientific evidence for the protective effects of vegetables on health is very strong. In coming weeks of the program, I'll give you other suggestions about enriching your diet with vegetables and recipes for preparing them.

The other dietary change I have asked you to make this week is to begin eating some fish if you do not already do so. The kinds of fish I have recommended are oily fish from cold, Northern waters: salmon, sardines, kippers, mackerel. Salmon is easily available fresh; the others you will find in cans. My reason for including these fish in the Eight-Week Program is that they are excellent sources of omega-3 fatty acids, special fats that have beneficial effects on many body functions. For example, they inhibit the clotting tendency of the blood, reducing the risk of heart attack. They improve the serum-lipid profile (blood fats), and they modify the production of hormones (eicosanoids; see page 117) that control tissue growth and repair, reducing excessive inflammation and promoting healing. If you do not want to eat fish, there are some vegetarian sources of omega-3s that I will tell you about in a moment, but be aware that including some fish in the diet may improve health in other ways. In general, fish-eating populations have higher longevity and lower rates of disease than non-fish-eating populations, and the differences may not have to do only with intake of omega-3 fatty acids.

I happen to like salmon a lot and will give you my favorite ways of preparing it at the end of this section (see page 54). Be aware that wild salmon is more nutritious, having a significantly higher content of omega-3s than farmed salmon. You can find canned kippers (smoked herring fillets) with or without added salt in all supermarkets. There are many preparations of sardines available as well. Avoid those packed in any oils other than sardine oil or olive oil; my preference is for water-packed ones. If you do get an oil-packed variety, drain off as much oil as you can before using the fish, in order to get rid of as many extra fat calories as you can. Fresh mackerel is delicious but available only seasonally; most stores stock canned mackerel fillets, sometimes in tomato—or another flavorful—sauce.

Here are your options for getting omega-3s in your diet without eating fish. You can buy capsules of fish oils in drugstores and health-food stores, but I advise you not to use them. It is not clear that they reproduce the benefits of whole fish, and they may contain toxic contaminants. Instead I suggest adding homemade flax meal to your diet, since this is a cheap and convenient source of the fatty acids you want. Buy whole flaxseeds at a natural-food store. Keep them in the refrigerator, and grind a half-cup or so at a time, using a blender or coffee grinder. Ground flax has a nutty taste that is quite good added to cereals, salads, potatoes, rice, or cooked vegetables. A tablespoon of the meal once a day will give you a good ration of omega-3s. Be aware that flaxseeds are high in fiber and will increase the bulk of stools; in some individuals they may exert a laxative effect. Most people find this effect welcome, but some do not. If it bothers you, eat less.

You will see dark plastic bottles of flaxseed oil in the refrigerator and freezer cases of natural-food stores. I think flax meal is preferable, being cheaper and tastier. Flax oil oxidizes very readily and, unless it is handled and packed with great care, develops the unpleasant taste of oil paint, a sign of rancidity and hardly a welcome addition to food. Other specialty oils that provide omega-3s but are not yet generally available come from the seeds of hemp and hops. Canola and soy oils are the only common vegetable oils that have omega-3s, though not nearly as much as flax.

There is also one vegetable that contains omega-3s: purslane (*Portulaca oleracea*), sometimes eaten as a wild green here but more commonly despised by gardeners as an invasive weed. In other parts of the world, people cultivate purslane and like it as a vegetable; Greeks often add it to soups, for example, and some experts think it contributes to the heart-healthiness of Mediterranean diets. Specialty seed catalogues offer improved varieties of purslane for home gardens. If you like to produce some of your own food, consider this easy-to-grow creeping plant with small, succulent leaves.

Here are some recipes to help you implement the dietary recommendations of this first week of the program:*

✌ *Broccoli* ✌

Here is my preferred preparation of this wonderfully healthful vegetable:

1 large bunch broccoli
1 tablespoon extra-virgin olive oil
salt to taste
several cloves garlic, chopped
red-pepper flakes to taste (optional)

1. Trim the bottoms of the broccoli stalks and discard. Cut off the main stem of each stalk, peel it to beneath the fibrous layer, and cut the flesh into edible chunks. Separate the head of broccoli into bite-size pieces and peel a bit of the skin from the small stems to make them more tender.

2. Wash the broccoli in cold water, drain it, and place in a pot with 1/4 cup cold water, the olive oil, salt to taste, and the garlic. Add a pinch or more of the hot red-pepper flakes if you want a spicy dish.

3. Bring to a boil, cover tightly, and let steam until the broccoli is bright green and very crunchy-tender, no more than 5 minutes. Remove with a slotted spoon and serve at once. You can also add the broccoli (with any remaining liquid) to cooked pasta (I prefer penne or rigatoni), seasoning with grated Parmesan cheese if you like.

---

* All recipes are meant to yield three to four servings, unless otherwise noted.

✌ *Grilled or Broiled Salmon* ✌

MARINADE
1 cup sake
1/2 cup natural soy sauce or tamari
1 tablespoon grated fresh gingerroot
2 cloves fresh garlic, mashed
1 tablespoon dark-brown sugar

salmon fillets (allow 6 ounces per person)
lemon wedges (optional)

1. Prepare the marinade by mixing the sake (Japanese rice wine), the natural soy sauce (a reduced-sodium variety if you prefer), the ginger, the garlic, and the dark-brown sugar.

2. Rinse the salmon fillets under cold water, place in a glass or ceramic dish, and pour the marinade over. Cover and let marinate in the refrigerator for 1–3 hours, spooning the liquid over any exposed parts of the fish once or twice.

3. Prepare the grill or preheat the broiler to high heat.

4. Drain the fish and place on foil on grill or rack in oven. Cook until desired doneness, but do not overcook. Serve at once, with lemon wedges if you like. Makes a great meal with rice and a cooked vegetable or salad.

✌ *Easy Poached Salmon* ✌

salmon fillets (allow 6 ounces per person)
1 carrot, sliced
1 small onion, sliced
1 stalk celery, sliced
2 slices lemon
several sprigs of parsley
6 bay leaves (Turkish if possible)
salt to taste
1 cup dry white wine
juice of half a lemon

1. Cut the salmon fillets into individual portions.

2. Place in a saucepan the carrot, onion, sliced celery, lemon, parsley, and bay leaves (Turkish, not California; if you have California bay leaves, use half of a large leaf).

3. Add the fish, cold water to cover, salt to taste, the wine, and the lemon juice. Bring the pot to a boil, uncovered.

4. Adjust heat to simmer and let fish cook for 5 minutes.

5. Turn off heat and leave fish undisturbed for 10 minutes. Then remove it carefully to a serving platter; the salmon will be perfectly done. It is delicious served either hot or cold.

✧ Salmon in Parchment ✧

This is an easy and elegant main-dish preparation. It requires cooking parchment, which you will find in rolls or sheets at kitchen-supply stores.

> *thin spaghetti*
> *olive oil*
> *salt*
> *fresh dill or parsley, chopped*
> *fresh vegetables (see procedure below)*
> *salmon fillet*
> *Dijon mustard*
> *baking parchment*

1. Heat oven to 400°F.

2. Cook thin spaghetti until just done (*al dente*), drain, toss with a bit of olive oil, salt, and chopped fresh dill (use parsley if dill is not available).

3. Prepare a garnish of fresh vegetables: carrot and zucchini matchsticks, asparagus tips, snow or snap pea pods, etc.

4. Rinse salmon fillet, cut in individual portions, and pat dry. Spread the top of each one with Dijon mustard.

5. For each person, place a serving of pasta on a sheet of parchment, top with a salmon fillet, add the vegetables, and twist the corners of the parchment together to seal into a pouch.

6. Place the pouches in the middle of the hot oven and bake for 10 minutes. Serve immediately in the sealed pouches, opening them just before eating.

๑๋ Dr. Andrew Weil's Favorite ๑๋
Low-Fat Salad Dressing

seasoned rice-wine vinegar (see note below)
dark-roasted sesame oil
1 clove garlic (optional)

Note: Seasoned rice-wine vinegar can be bought in a Japanese grocery store or the Asian-food section of a supermarket; it is seasoned with sugar and salt. Avoid brands that contain MSG (monosodium glutamate). You can also buy plain rice-wine vinegar and season it yourself with sugar or honey and salt to taste.

1. Pour enough vinegar over prepared salad greens in a serving bowl to coat them lightly.
2. Add a teaspoon of dark-roasted sesame oil—its flavor is so intense that a little goes a remarkably long way.
3. Toss well and serve.

This couldn't be easier. For variety, you can try adding a clove of garlic, crushed, to the vinegar before you pour it over the greens.

Supplements

You are to start taking vitamin C this week, the first of four antioxidant supplements making up a formula that I take myself and recommend for everyone. Maybe you already take vitamin C and other dietary supplements. If you do not, here are the reasons to begin doing so.

Almost all animals make vitamin C in their bodies. Only human beings, other primates, and a very few other species have lost this ability and need to get the vitamin every day from dietary sources, principally fresh fruits and vegetables. You need certain levels of vitamin C to build strong connective tissue, including the linings of coronary arteries, and to allow the healing system to repair wounds. I believe that higher doses can encourage healing on all levels as well as help the body protect itself from oxidative damage by free radicals, the highly reactive molecules generated by exposure to chemical and energetic toxins as well as by normal metabolism.

As an example of vitamin C's effect on the healing system, let me tell a story that happened just a few weeks ago. The older brother of a friend of mine underwent surgery for removal of portions of his stomach and esophagus. Before he entered the hospital, he asked me what he could do to speed his recovery, and I gave him two standard recommendations. First, I told him to get permission from the anesthesiologist to wear a headset during the operation and have an audiotape made of suggestions for success of the surgery and a rapid recovery with minimal pain. This would serve two purposes: it would block out any conversations in the operating room that put unwanted ideas in his mind, and it would take advantage of the mind's influence on the healing system in a state when the unconscious mind readily accepts suggestion. My second recommendation was to tell his surgeon that he wanted high doses of vitamin C put into his intravenous drip from the time he went into surgery until the IV was removed: 20 grams in every twenty-four-hour period. I also told him not to expect compliance with this request; in my experience, most hospitals will not honor it.

This patient took a very aggressive stance with his doctors and insisted on the intravenous vitamin C. He got it. When the surgeon examined him several days after the operation, he told the patient that he had never seen such rapid healing from a surgical wound and was so impressed that he would begin ordering IV vitamin C in all of his cases.

Supplemental vitamin C is nontoxic. It does not promote the formation of kidney stones, as some have charged, but it can disturb bowel function in very high dosage. If you take increasing doses of this vitamin, you will at some point reach your level of bowel tolerance, marked initially by flatulence and then by diarrhea. You will want to stay below the dose that causes these effects, and since the level varies greatly from person to person, you may have to experiment. I recommend 1 to 2 grams (1,000 to 2,000 milligrams) two to three times a day, for a total daily dose of 2 to 6 grams (2,000 to 6,000 milligrams). If you can remember to take this vitamin three times a day (say, at breakfast, dinner, and bedtime), that will keep it available to your body all the time. At least try to take it twice a day, at twelve-hour intervals.

I like to use an effervescent, powdered form of vitamin C that is nonacidic. (See the appendix for a source.) Do not use sweet, chewable tablets (bad for the teeth) or huge, hard tablets (may not dissolve), or fancy brands that are very expensive. Do not expect immediate effects from vitamin C, although it may decrease frequency of colds and reduce easy bruising in some people. You are taking it as part of a long-range strategy to protect your healing system and enhance its functioning so it will be able to maintain your day-to-day well-being and be ready to serve you in case of illness.

Exercise

Exercise is a key component of a healthy lifestyle. You cannot enjoy optimal health and healing if you are sedentary. You may have heard that walking is the best exercise. It's true, and I'm asking you to do a lot of it in this Eight-Week Program. Here are the advantages of walking:

- You already know how to do it.
- You can do it anywhere.
- It requires no equipment, just a good pair of shoes.
- It carries the least risk of injury of any form of exercise.
- It can provide a complete workout, equal to or better than any other activity.
- It will satisfy all your exercise requirements throughout your life, even into old age.

Many fitness buffs look down on walking as being tame compared with running, playing competitive sports, or driving oneself to sweaty exhaustion on stationary bicycles and other aerobic torture devices. It's not so. I have seen people attain maximum fitness through walking alone; they did it conscientiously and regularly and did enough of it to take full advantage of its wonderful conditioning effect on the body, and they used no other form of physical activity to get to their goal. I have also seen very obese people reach their optimal weights in several months by walking every day in combination with sensible dietary modification (see pages 235–40 for details).

My preference is to walk outside in beautiful surroundings, but if I'm in a city, I will gladly walk around it as much as possible, and if I encounter bad weather, I might just walk back and forth in a shopping mall or try to find a gym where I can walk on a treadmill. For maximum cardiovascular benefit, you should try to include some uphill walking—long, moderate, sustained grades are terrific—or walk fast enough to get your heart rate up.* Sometimes I like to walk alone and be with my thoughts and nature. Sometimes I like to walk with a friend and pass the time in conversation. Sometimes I carry a portable cassette player and listen to spirited music with a beat that keeps my feet moving quickly. Cassette players and tapes have transformed walking for many; I know people who like to listen to books-on-tape or foreign-language lessons while they do their daily walks.

I've asked you to begin this practice with a ten-minute daily walk (if you are already walking this much or more, keep at it!), and I want you to do it even if you have some other exercise routine, because I feel that walking offers benefits that other forms of activity do not, such as conditioning rhythms in the brain in response to the coordinated motions of the arms and legs. If you are not used to walking, be sure to wear the right shoes. I recommend running shoes with good cushioning in the insole; many brands are available at athletic-supply stores. You will also find special double-layer socks that prevent blisters and wick away perspiration from your feet. Think about where you are going to walk and when, how you are going to build this activity into your daily routine. I like to take morning walks, before breakfast, but if I miss the chance, I'm just as happy to walk at the end of the day.

In the next few weeks, as walking time increases, I will give you more information about this key component of the Eight-Week Program.

Mental/Spiritual

The recommendations that fall under this heading are most important. If you have read my earlier writings on health, you know that I am a strong proponent of mind/body medicine who believes that illness in the physical body is often the result of imbalance in the mind

---

* You can buy a miniature heart-rate monitor to wear like a wristwatch (along with a band that straps around your chest), or you can learn to take your pulse at the wrist for fifteen seconds and multiply by four to get beats per minute. The Target Heart Rate Zone (THRZ), in which maximal aerobic conditioning takes place and fat burning occurs, can be calculated by a not-too-complicated formula. First determine your Predicted Maximal Heart Rate (PMHR). For physically inactive men and women of any activity level, the PMHR is 220 minus your age; for physically active men it is 205 minus your age. THRZ is then 65 to 75 percent of your PMHR. For example, I am now 54 and physically active, so my PMHR is 151. My THRZ is 98–113, and a fifteen-second pulse rate in this zone would be one-quarter of those figures, or 24–28. In general, if you are exercising above your THRZ, you will be too aerobically stressed to carry on a conversation, and if you are exercising below it, you will not notice your heart and breath going significantly faster than normal.

or the spiritual realm. For your healing system to function optimally, you must address those areas of your being as well as look after the needs of your body. I will ease you into this area of work with practices that are gentle and interesting, that I think you will enjoy, and that, despite their simplicity, are profoundly effective.

This week, I have asked you to think about your own experiences of healing—from any recent illnesses, injuries, or problems (emotional as well as physical). I want you to focus attention on healing, because the way to experience more of something you want is to become more conscious of it. If you like to keep journals or diaries, you might want to get a notebook in which to record these experiences and new ones. It is a way to build up confidence in the power of spontaneous healing inside you.

Next, I have asked you to begin working with your breath, a practice that will develop as you progress through the Eight-Week Program. I have written extensively about the healing power of breath in other books. Suffice it to say that breath is the link between the body and mind and between the conscious and unconscious mind. It is the master key to the control of emotions and to the operations of the involuntary nervous system. Moreover, breath represents the movement of spirit in matter. Turning your attention to your breath moves you naturally toward relaxation and meditation and puts you in conscious touch with your vital, nonphysical essence.

The very simplest technique of breath work is simply to observe it, to do nothing other than follow the breath cycle with your observing mind, without trying to influence it in any way. Here are the formal instructions:

1. Sit in a comfortable position with your back straight and your eyes lightly closed, having loosened any tight clothing.
2. Focus your attention on your breathing, and follow the contours of the cycle through inhalation and exhalation, noting, if you can, the points at which one phase changes into the other.

Do this for five minutes once a day. Your goal is simply to keep your attention on the breath cycle and observe. No matter how the breath changes, even if the excursions become very small, just continue to follow them. This is a basic form of meditation, a relaxation method, and a way to begin to harmonize body, mind, and spirit.

Finally, this week I have asked you to buy some fresh flowers to keep in your home, where you can enjoy them. I do not think much commentary is required. Flowers manifest the beauty and wonder of nature and delight the senses. It feels good to be around them. They raise our spirits.

That is all the information you need to go through the first week of the Eight-Week Program.

A Healing Story:
The Value of Supplements

Here is a short, happy story from Patti Lewis of Tempe, Arizona:

I have followed your recommendations for vitamins and nutrients. By doing so my recovery from breast cancer was a positive, healing experience. Breast cancer forever changed my life. Before the diagnosis I never gave much thought or effort to building up my immune system. I was healthy, so it wasn't important. Now I take very good care of myself and follow your practical, commonsense approach to good health.

The supplements kept me healthy throughout the cold-and-flu season even though my immune system had been zapped by chemotherapy. They played a key role in keeping my mind, body, and spirit in balance. My spirits remained high as I recovered, and I was able to find humor in everything. I continued riding my bike as I recovered, which kept me fit and happy. Friends and family would shake their heads and marvel at how well I did. Your recommendations were worth their weight in gold. I will continue on the supplements and look forward to a long, healthy, and happy life.

6

WEEK TWO

Projects

• Find out where your drinking water comes from if you do not know, and what impurities it might contain. Stop drinking chlorinated water. Get information on a water-purifying system for your home, if you do not have one. In the meantime, buy bottled water.

Diet

• Again eat fish at least once this week and broccoli twice.
• Try to increase your consumption of whole grains. Choose whole-grain breads or cereals, for example. Or try any of the recipes for grain dishes you will find here (beginning on page 72).
• Go to a natural-food store and look through the frozen and refrigerated sections to familiarize yourself with the many different products made from soybeans. Select one to try.
• Buy some Japanese or Chinese green tea and try it. If you drink coffee or black tea, try to substitute green tea for some or all of your usual beverage.

Supplements

• Start taking one capsule a day of mixed carotenes with breakfast. The product should provide 25,000 IU (international units) of beta-carotene along with related compounds (like alpha-carotene, lutein,

and zeaxanthin). It must contain lycopene to give you the full benefits of this family of natural pigments.

Exercise

• Increase your daily walk to fifteen minutes.

Mental/Spiritual

• Visit a park or some other favorite place in nature. Spend as much
time as you can there, doing nothing in particular, just feeling the energy of the place.
• Try a one-day "news fast." Do not read, watch, or listen to any
news for a day.
• Continue with Breath Observation for five minutes a day and add
a second breathing exercise: for one minute a day, try to experience
the breath cycle beginning with exhalation and ending with inhalation. Details of the "Begin with Exhalation" exercise are given on
pages 78–9.

Optional

• Pay attention to your mental imagery and make a few notes on the
kinds of images that have strong emotional impact on you. Think
about how you might adapt them to use in healing visualizations.

COMMENTARY

Projects

Drinking water is one of the major sources of environmental toxins
that can harm your healing system; fortunately, it is one that you can
do something about.

    According to recent reports, drinking water in the U.S. is increas-
ingly becoming a health risk, whether you live in a big city or a rural
area. More than one hundred million Americans drink water that
contains significant levels of three cancer-causing chemicals: arsenic,
radon, and chlorine by-products (trihalomethanes, or THMs). Ni-

trates—which can cause deadly "blue-baby syndrome" when infant formula is made with tap water polluted by it—has been found at excessive levels in more than two thousand water systems in forty states; rural areas with significant agricultural runoff are in the most danger.

In addition to chemical contamination, chlorine-resistant viruses and parasites such as *Cryptosporidium* and *Giardia* can slip through the more than one thousand large water systems in this country lacking proper filters. (According to the Centers for Disease Control, almost a million people become sick in the U.S. each year from waterborne micro-organisms.) In my opinion, chlorine is itself a major health risk and should be phased out in favor of safer methods of disinfection, like ozonation. Besides forming THMs when it reacts with organic compounds, chlorine by itself is a strong oxidizing agent that may promote coronary heart disease and damage body defenses.

Despite the degraded quality of our drinking water, laws on this matter are inadequate, and enforcement of them is weak. "Safe" levels of contamination are simply set too high, and not enough of the proven contaminants are regulated (only sixty of the seven hundred dangerous chemicals found regularly in our drinking water). The Environmental Protection Agency (EPA) does not yet require monitoring of radioactive materials, heavy metals, chlorine by-products, or *Cryptosporidium*. Furthermore, water suppliers routinely fail to notify customers when water is found to be contaminated, even though the law requires them to do so.

Here are my suggestions for what to do, given the situation we face:

• Never drink water that tastes of chlorine, even if it means going thirsty. Order bottled water if you are out, or carry a portable carbon filter (see appendix for a source) that filters a glass at a time, removing chlorine and other bad tastes.

• If you buy water from a water company, ask for the results of the tests that companies are required to make available. If you are on a private system, have your water tested annually by a laboratory (see appendix). You want to know whether fecal-coliform bacteria, lead, fluorine, chlorine, arsenic, nitrates, and hardness fall within safe levels, as well as whether the water contains parasites, other micro-organisms, sulfates, herbicides, pesticides, and any other contaminants that might occur in your area. Use water drawn from your tap, so any pollutants such as lead that may be leaching from your pipes will be detected. Test the water at a different time each year, since some pollutants, like nitrates, may be present only seasonally. Only the results of water testing can tell you whether you need to buy a purifying system and if so what kind.

• If you get water from a municipal system, be sure to test your tap water for lead, because plumbing inside the house is the major source of lead contamination, and this will not show up in the municipal tests. Water containing more than ten parts per billion of lead is a health risk, especially for infants, children, and pregnant women, but probably for everyone else as well.

• Flush your pipes daily by letting water run for three to five minutes in the morning, or after any periods of disuse, before drinking any or using it to prepare food. "First-draw" water, because of possible higher concentration of lead and other contaminants, is more dangerous.

• Never use hot tap water for drinking or cooking. It is unfit for human consumption, because impurities from plumbing and the insides of hot-water tanks more readily leach out through it.

• Bottled water is, at best, a temporary solution to the drinking-water problem. It is much too expensive for regular use, and you cannot count on its safety. Much bottled water is tap water in disguise, and even bottled spring water can be contaminated. (In 1990, for example, benzene—an organic solvent—was found in some bottles of carbonated Perrier water.) Cleanliness is the biggest concern, because bacteria can breed quickly in unchlorinated water. In one EPA check of twenty-five bottling plants, serious problems with cleanliness were found at every one.

• If you use bottled water, ask the manufacturer for information about the source of the water and the results of testing. When you find a reliable source, have the water delivered directly to your home, or buy it at stores that have good turnover. Keep the water out of sunlight and use it quickly. To minimize chemical contamination from containers, get water in glass or clear plastic jugs—not the soft, translucent plastic ones, whose material leaches into the water.

• A home purifying system is a good investment in your health, but if you need one—based on the results of water tests—you must do some homework to decide what kind you require. You may be able to get by with a simple device that removes bad tastes and odors, but you will probably need a system that uses more than one technology to remove organic chemicals, heavy metals, nitrates, and bacteria.

• Don't rely on free tests offered by the companies selling purifiers—they are not thorough enough. Use an independent laboratory.

• See the appendix for sources of information on types of water purifiers, and only buy a system that meets the standards of the National Sanitation Foundation (NSF).

• At this writing, one of the best and most affordable systems uses a combination of two technologies: carbon-block filtration and an electrochemical method that exposes water to a copper-zinc alloy called KDF. Under-the-counter systems of this sort cost less than $500 and are easy to maintain. They remove most of the worrisome contaminants (although you may have to add another component to remove nitrates if you live in an area with high agricultural runoff), and KDF puts trace amounts of copper and zinc into the water, which most experts consider beneficial.

• Buy a system with standard-sized cartridges, so that you will be able to get replacement parts even if the manufacturer goes out of business. Also choose a system based on the per-gallon cost of the purified water, not on the initial cost. Some systems cost less at first but are expensive to operate because of energy usage and replacement parts.

• If you get an under-the-counter model, get a stainless-steel faucet, not one made of brass-lead alloy, which can leach lead into the water.

• Know the maintenance schedule of your system and adhere to it. Filters eventually become exhausted, and bacteria can build up in some systems. Consider buying a meter so you can base cartridge replacements on the number of gallons purified rather than on some time limit.

• If you purify your water, you may have to rely on fluoride supplements to protect your teeth; ask your dentist about this.

It may seem that I've written too many words on this subject, but I've done it to impress you with the importance of protecting yourself and your healing system from toxins. Those in our food and in the air are not so easy to deal with. Water we can all do something about.

Diet

Whole grains, containing the germ and bran as well as the starch of staple seed crops, are excellent sources of fiber, which is generally deficient in our diets. Fiber keeps the digestive system running well, helps lower cholesterol, reduces risk of colon cancer, slows absorption of sugar into the bloodstream, and probably does many other good things for our bodies as well, even if researchers do not yet know the details and mechanisms. It is recommended that people eat 40 grams of fiber a day, twice what most of us consume. White flour provides very little of it; you would have to eat fifty loaves of white bread to get your recommended daily allowance from that source alone.

The best way to get more fiber is simply to eat more fresh vegetables and fruits as well as products made from whole grains. Many good-tasting whole-grain breakfast cereals are available, both hot and cold, as well as a variety of whole grains that make excellent alternatives to white rice. You can now buy red rice and black rice in addition to short- and long-grain brown rice, as well as buckwheat groats (kasha), quinoa, and wild rice (now cultivated extensively and much more affordable than it used to be). You don't have to exclude white bread and other refined-flour products from your life. Just eat fewer of them and more whole-grain products along with your vegetables and fruit.

This week I want you also to learn about the wonders of soybeans. For centuries the Chinese and Japanese have cultivated soy as a dietary staple, an excellent source of protein that can be turned into multitudinous edibles, from a kind of milk and cheese to foods that are exact facsimiles of animal foods that were prohibited in some Buddhist traditions. Only recently have Westerners begun to discover the delights of soy foods, and only very recently have Western researchers begun to take notice of the contribution of these foods to the low incidence of Western diseases in parts of Asia.

Besides being cheaper, soybeans are better than animal foods in several ways. Their protein does not come with a load of saturated fat that will stimulate your liver to make cholesterol, and they provide your digestive tract with fiber. They also contain *isoflavones,* unusual compounds that may offer significant protection against cancer. These appear to interact with estrogen receptors in the human body, and for that reason researchers also call them *phytoestrogens,* meaning plant-derived estrogenlike substances.

A number of diseases in women are estrogenically driven—that is, they result from increased production of or exposure to estrogenic hormones, with resultant overgrowth or abnormal growth of cells that respond to them. Fibrocystic changes in breasts, breast cancer, uterine cancer, uterine fibroids, and endometriosis are examples of such diseases. Some of these ailments, breast cancer in particular, are increasing at alarming rates throughout the world.

One theory explains the rise in terms of increased exposure of women to *xenoestrogens*—foreign estrogens, not those made by a woman's own ovaries. It is well known that estrogenic hormones are used as growth promoters in animals raised commercially for food; residues of these hormones find their way into beef, pork, poultry, and dairy products, unless the foods are certified to be free of such chemicals. But a more disturbing possibility is that the environment may be saturated with pollutants that act as xenoestrogens, which enter our bodies and push receptive cells in the direction of increased division and growth and increased risk of malignant transformation. A number of industrial by-products and pesticides fall into this category; they are now widespread in soil and water.

You can do only so much to prevent these toxins from entering your body, but the phytoestrogens in soybeans offer a sound defensive strategy: they may be able to occupy estrogen receptors, activating them only weakly but blocking access by the stronger foreign estrogens. Japanese women on traditional diets had very low rates of breast cancer. (I say "had" because the traditional diet is rapidly becoming a thing of the past, as meat and other Western foods become tremendously popular in Japan.) When Japanese women moved to America and ate American diets, their breast-cancer rate rapidly rose to equal that of their American counterparts. Medical researchers used to think it was dietary fat that made the difference—the traditional Japanese diet is one of the lowest in fat in the world, whereas Americans get more than a third of their calories from fat—but recent studies cast doubt on the importance of high fat intake as a major risk factor for breast cancer.

I think the prominence of soy foods in Japan is more likely to be the key difference. Japanese women also have much less trouble with menopausal symptoms than American women, probably because they get protective phytoestrogens in their diet. And there is reason to think that these compounds afford men protection from prostate cancer, another hormonally driven malignancy (driven, in this case, by androgens—male sex hormones—which are antagonized by estrogens). Two of the best-studied soy isoflavones are genistein and daidzein. Recently, I've seen these compounds offered for sale in health-food stores in pill form, hyped as being the pure magic of soybeans that protects people from cancer. As in the case of sulphoraphane ("broccoli in a pill"), this is just another instance of reductionist thinking: the part is equal to the whole. Whole soybeans and many foods made from them seem to be anticarcinogenic; it is foolish to think that an isolated component reproduces this effect.

A favorite snack in Japan is fresh whole green soybeans—known as *edamame*—boiled in their pods in salted water, served cold as appetizers at sushi bars, and eaten at home with beer, much as we eat peanuts in the shell. You pick up a pod and pop the tasty beans directly into your mouth. Traditionally, these were available only in Japan in summer, but I now see frozen *edamame* in Asian grocery stores here, and you can get them year-round. Please try them. I think you will find them very appealing.

In my opinion, one of the healthiest dietary changes people can make is to substitute soy foods for some (or all) of the animal foods they now eat. To start this process, you need to become familiar with the range of choices available, which is why I ask you this week to do some looking through a natural-food store. You will find tofu, tempeh, soy wieners and burgers, lunch "meats," and many other products. Some of these are excellent, some are terrible; you can eat some right out of the package, others require preparation. For example, tofu is an extremely versatile food, but you cannot just take it home, dump it into a salad, and expect your family to like it. With a little ingenuity and effort, it can be turned into delicious main dishes, spreads, even desserts that do not seem strange at all. The new generation of soy burgers now in stores are so meatlike in appearance and taste that some vegetarians refuse to eat them. Please experiment.

Let me give you a few cautions about soy foods. Some—especially soy grits, soy flour, and texturized vegetable protein (TVP)—can cause terrific flatulence if you are not used to them. In general, these ingredients predominate in old-style soy foods that have been around for years, mostly eaten by groups like Seventh-Day Adventists, who shun meat. The new kinds of soy foods do not cause this problem. Be aware also that soybeans are high in fat. The fat is polyunsaturated and not harmful from a cardiovascular perspective, which makes substituting soy foods for animal foods a heart-healthy move. Nonetheless, it can add too many fat calories to your diet. Look for reduced-fat tofu, and check the fat content of processed foods. Some of the best soy wieners and burgers come in completely fat-free versions that are very tasty. Note that the highly processed products made with "isolated soy protein" may not deliver the anticancer isoflavones. As consumers become more aware of their benefits, manufacturers may begin to add them back, and labels may come to state content of genistein and daidzein. Finally, whenever possible, try to buy products made from organically grown soybeans.

Once you find some soy foods that you like, I'm going to ask you to substitute them for some of the animal foods in your diet.

The other experiment I have asked you to conduct this week is to buy and drink some Japanese or Chinese green tea. Green tea is the unfermented leaf of the tea plant, *Camellia sinensis*. In the preparation of the more familiar black tea, leaves are piled up in heaps and briefly "sweated," a natural fermentation process that darkens the leaves and changes their aroma and flavor. Recently, medical researchers have discovered a number of health benefits of tea, having to do with its content of polyphenols (catechins). Green tea provides more catechins than black tea, because some of these compounds are destroyed during sweating. (Oolong tea falls in between, having a color, flavor, and catechin content intermediate between green and black tea.) Catechins lower cholesterol and improve lipid metabolism. They also have significant anticancer and antibacterial effects. As news of these remarkable properties of green tea has spread, health-food stores have begun to sell it in pill form, which my Japanese friends find laughable. There are even green-tea underarm deodorants that rely on its antibacterial properties.

All tea contains theophylline, a close relative of caffeine, and a natural stimulant. People can become addicted to tea but not nearly so readily as to coffee. In moderation—say, one to two cups a day—green tea, with its delicate aroma and slightly bitter taste, makes a pleasant and healthful addition to the diet. Many grades and qualities of it exist, so shop around to see what pleases you. You will find green-tea bags in some supermarkets, but for a more interesting selection, go to Asian grocery stores or any of the specialty tea shops that are now growing in popularity.

If you drink coffee or cola, try substituting tea. If you already drink black tea, try substituting green. If you do not currently take any caffeine, consider drinking some decaffeinated tea, which still has its catechins. You may even be able to find a decaffeinated form of green tea. Be aware that the ordinary tea bags that most Americans are used to contain distinctly inferior grades of black tea. It is worth investing some time and effort to discover good-quality tea that you can enjoy. I learned to drink green tea in Japan and associate it with good times there; when I inhale its subtle fragrance, I am transported to tatami rooms in temples and country inns, where I sat on the floor with friends, admiring flower arrangements and artfully served food. The experience is sensual and meditative at the same time, and I know that I am giving my body something that is good for it.

Now here are some recipes for you to try out this week:

✎ *Kasha with Vegetables* ✎

This recipe features buckwheat groats (kasha), a grainlike staple of northern Europe and Russia. It is easier to make the dish with toasted buckwheat groats; if you can only find raw ones, you can toast them lightly in a dry skillet over medium heat, stirring frequently.

2 ounces dried mushrooms
1 cup buckwheat groats (kasha)
1 large carrot, sliced
1 medium onion, coarsely chopped
salt or natural soy sauce to taste

1. Soak the dried mushrooms (shiitake or porcini are very flavorful) in water until soft. Drain, saving the soaking water, and slice, discarding any tough portions.

2. Add the groats to 3 cups of boiling water (including the mushroom-soaking liquid), lower heat, and add the carrot, the onion, and the mushrooms.

3. Cover and simmer until water is absorbed. Add salt or natural soy sauce to taste.

ᴖ Easy Miso Soup ᴕ

Miso is a traditional fermented-soybean product used every day in Japanese cooking. You will find many varieties of natural miso in the refrigerated cases of health-food stores, both stronger-flavored dark ones and milder light ones. All are good and keep indefinitely under refrigeration. This soup gives you the benefits of soybeans along with vegetables and ginger.

> *2 teaspoons canola oil*
> *3 slices fresh gingerroot*
> *1 large onion, thinly sliced*
> *2 carrots, thinly sliced*
> *2 stalks celery, thinly sliced*
> *4 cups coarsely chopped cabbage*
> *4 tablespoons miso*
> *2 scallions, very thinly sliced*
> *dark-roasted sesame oil to taste*

1. Heat the canola oil in a large pot.

2. Add the ginger and the onion; sauté over medium heat for 5 minutes.

3. Add the carrots, celery, and cabbage. Stir well.

4. Add 5 cups water, bring rapidly to a boil, then lower heat and simmer, covered, until vegetables are just tender, about 10 minutes. Remove from heat.

5. Place the miso in a bowl, add a little of the broth, and stir well to a smooth cream. Add more broth to thin the mixture, then add it to the pot of soup. Let rest for a few minutes.

6. Serve in bowls with the raw scallions. You may wish to remove the ginger slices before serving, and you can add a few drops of the sesame oil to each bowl if desired.

ᴖ Tofu Salad or Sandwich Filling ᴕ

> *1-pound block tofu*
> *1 teaspoon ground turmeric*
> *1 tablespoon prepared mustard*

1 tablespoon sweet pickle relish
3 tablespoons chopped celery
3 tablespoons chopped onion
1 tablespoon chopped fresh parsley
dash paprika
salt to taste
hot-pepper sauce or salsa (optional)

1. Drain the tofu well and mash it roughly in a bowl.
2. Add the turmeric, mustard, sweet pickle relish, celery, onion, parsley, paprika, and salt to taste.
3. Mix and mash well. Correct seasoning. Add hot-pepper sauce or salsa to taste.

↶ Vegetable Stir-Fry with Tofu ↷

1 pound baked, pressed tofu
8 cups sliced vegetables: onions, carrots, peppers, mushrooms, celery,
broccoli, asparagus, mung-bean sprouts (substitutions allowed)
1 tablespoon canola oil

FLAVORING MIXTURE
1/4 cup dry sherry
1/4 cup natural soy sauce
2 cloves garlic, mashed
2 tablespoons light-brown sugar
1 teaspoon finely chopped gingerroot
1 teaspoon dark-roasted sesame oil

Note: Baked, pressed tofu is available refrigerated in health-food stores and Asian grocery stores.

1. Slice the tofu into strips and arrange on a plate with prepared vegetables, separated by variety. (In many supermarkets you can now find loose or packaged mixtures of vegetables ready for stir-frying.)
2. Add the canola oil to a large skillet or wok, place over medium-high heat, and add vegetables. Cook sturdier vegetables first, saving tender ones like bean sprouts and asparagus for later. Stir vegetables

constantly, adding a little water if necessary to keep them from sticking or burning. The idea is to produce a mixture in which all the items are crunchy-tender and retain their colors and individual character.

3. Add the tofu and the flavoring mixture (which has been stirred together till the sugar dissolves). Continue to cook over high heat for 1 minute, then serve over rice or noodles.

❧ Grilled Tempeh Sandwiches ❧

Tempeh is another fermented-soybean product, a staple food of Indonesia, with a meaty texture and a bland flavor. You will find packages of it refrigerated or frozen in health-food stores.

1 package tempeh

MARINADE
1 cup red wine
4 tablespoons olive oil
3 large garlic cloves, mashed
2 teaspoons coriander seeds, crushed (or 1 teaspoon ground coriander)
salt to taste

bread
lettuce and tomato, sliced

1. Thaw tempeh if frozen and cut the cakes in half crosswise, then split each half horizontally, using a long sharp knife.
2. Marinate the tempeh slices at least 1 hour at room temperature or 3 hours in the refrigerator.
3. Drain the tempeh and grill or broil until well browned. Make sandwiches of it on toasted bread with lettuce, tomato, and your favorite spread.

❧ Apple–Oat Bran Muffins ❧

2 cups whole-wheat pastry flour
1 cup unbleached white flour
1 1/4 cups oat bran

2 1/2 teaspoons baking soda
1 teaspoon cinnamon
1/4 teaspoon nutmeg
1 12-ounce can frozen pure apple-juice concentrate, thawed
2 large green cooking apples, peeled and coarsely chopped

1. Heat oven to 325°F. and lightly oil a muffin tin.

2. In a bowl, sift together the pastry flour, white flour, oat bran, baking soda, cinnamon, and nutmeg. Add the apple-juice concentrate, the chopped apples, and enough water (about 1 cup) to make a light batter. Mix just enough to moisten all ingredients.

3. Divide batter among 12 cups of muffin tin and bake until lightly browned, 25–30 minutes. Remove muffins from cups while hot.

ﾍ Quinoa Pudding ﾍ

Here is an unusual, healthy dessert made from the staple grain-like seed of the high Andes, now available in specialty food shops and health-food stores.

1 cup quinoa
2 cups apple juice
1 cup raisins
1 cup chopped nuts
juice of 1 lemon
cinnamon to taste
salt to taste
2 teaspoons vanilla extract
berries, sliced banana, or maple syrup (optional)

1. Place the quinoa in a sieve and wash it well under cold running water. Drain and place in pot with 2 cups cold water. Bring to a boil, cover, lower heat, and boil gently until all the water is absorbed, and quinoa is tender, about 15 minutes.

2. Measure 2 cups cooked quinoa and to it add the apple juice, raisins, nuts, lemon juice, and pinches of cinnamon and salt to taste. Simmer, covered, for 15 minutes.

3. Remove from heat and stir in the vanilla extract.

4. Chill. Serve plain, or with berries or sliced banana or a little maple syrup if you want it sweeter.

Supplements

The mixed-carotene supplement that I ask you to begin taking this week is the second component of the antioxidant formula that will protect your healing system. Fruits and vegetables that contain carotenes, a family of red and orange pigments related to vitamin A, have great cancer-protective value. These include cantaloupes, peaches, apricots, mangoes, squashes, and sweet potatoes; dark leafy greens like collards and kale; and, of course, carrots. Until recently, many health professionals advised people to take supplements of beta-carotene, one of the principal members of the carotene family and a direct precursor of vitamin A, but new research has cast doubt on the ability of beta-carotene alone to reproduce the protective effect of foods that contain it.

To suppose that beta-carotene is a carrot in a pill is more of the same kind of misguided thinking that I have noted above in reference to supplements of sulphoraphane from broccoli and genistein from soy. Nonetheless, many studies in the medical literature document the usefulness of beta-carotene as an antioxidant, particularly when it is taken with vitamin C and the rest of the complete formula. New products are available that combine it with some of the other carotenoid pigments, and I believe these are much better. One of the lesser-known carotenoids, lycopene, the red pigment in tomatoes, was recently reported to reduce the risk of prostate cancer. Taking a mixed-carotene supplement does not excuse you from eating tomatoes, carrots, and greens, but it is useful insurance against failing to supply your body with all the dietary carotenes it needs to protect itself from toxic damage and the effects of aging.

Read labels carefully to make sure the product you buy includes lycopene and gives you 25,000 IU of beta-carotene.

Exercise

You are increasing your daily walks to fifteen minutes. Try to make them brisk enough to increase your heart rate and breathing, perhaps by going up a hill. I want you to walk at least five days this week. Remember, this is the best all-around conditioning treatment you can give your body.

Mental/Spiritual

Connecting with nature is healing. It slows us down, takes us out of our routines, and reminds us that we live on a remarkable planet that we share with many other forms of life. Walking or sitting quietly in a natural setting is a simple form of meditation, an antidote for being too much in our heads, too focused on thoughts and emotions. If you live in a big city, seek out a park to visit. You will find the air better there and the trees comforting. You do not have to do anything in particular, just sit quietly and let the place relax you. Maybe you already have a favorite spot to go to, or maybe you would like to explore this week to discover a new one.

I have also asked you to try a one-day news fast this week. I do not want you to become uninformed about the state of the world, but I note that paying attention to news commonly results in anxiety, rage, and other emotional states that probably impede the healing system. I have given you many suggestions about diet, about nourishing your body. I think it is useful to broaden the concept of nutrition to include what we put into our consciousness as well. Many people do not exercise much control over that and as a result take in a lot of mental junk food. My goal in asking you to practice news fasting throughout the Eight-Week Program is for you to discover that you have the power to decide how much of this material you want to let in. I have no objection to your turning on the news for information you really need; I worry about people who turn it on compulsively or unconsciously, who are addicted to the news and the emotional ups and downs it provides. Observe any difference you feel in your state of mind and body when you opt to ignore the news. Are you less anxious? less stressed? less angry? less fearful? When you get to the end of the Eight-Week Program, I will ask you again, and at that time you can decide how much news you want to let back into your life.

Finally, I want you to add a second breathing exercise to your routine of Breath Observation from last week. This one is called "Begin with Exhalation," and I think you will find it interesting.

Breathing is continuous, with no beginning or end, but we tend to think of one breath as beginning with an inhalation and ending with an exhalation. I want you to practice reversing this perception. Try it at the end of the five minutes of Breath Observation. Again, focus attention on the breath without trying to influence it, but now experience exhalation as the beginning of each new cycle. Do this for just one minute. I think you will be surprised to find how different breathing is when you stand it on its head in this way. When I begin with exhalation, I find myself much more involved with my breath, actively working with it rather than passively experiencing it.

There is an important physiological reason for asking you to make this reversal: potentially you have greater control over exhalation than inhalation, because you can use the voluntary muscles between your ribs (the intercostal muscles) to squeeze air out of your lungs, and this musculature is much more powerful than that used for drawing air in. When you move more air out, you will automatically take more air in. It is desirable to deepen respiration, and the easiest way to do that is to start thinking of exhalation as the first part of the cycle and not worry at all about inhaling. By the way, the Chinese character for "breath" has two components, one meaning "exhalation," the other "inhalation," and exhalation comes first.

Keep in mind that the breathing exercises are an integral and unique aspect of the Eight-Week Program. Breath is a master key to health and healing, and I want you to learn how to make full use of it. I am often asked, "If you could only tell people to do one thing that would give them greater access to spontaneous healing, what would it be?" I never hesitate in answering, "Work with your breath!"

Optional

I have written elsewhere about visualization as a powerful technique to gain access to healing. Hypnotherapy, guided-imagery therapy, and other variations on the theme all take advantage of visual imagination as a key to the mind/body connection. In my experience, no part of the body or disease process is beyond the reach of these approaches. In some cases, visualization can produce complete healing responses; in others, it can boost the effectiveness and mitigate the toxicity of conventional therapies. To increase the chance of its working, you must use images that have strong emotional resonance. It is not enough to have someone tell you to bathe your body in white light. You are much more likely to activate your healing system if you use emotionally charged images, whether you take them from nature, computer graphics, or sexual fantasy. Only you know what kinds of images elicit a gut-level response from you; it is worth taking an inventory of your mental imagery to find the pictures that do it. Note them down and think about how you might employ them if you ever need to use visualization to help yourself deal with an illness or injury.

A Healing Story:
Seeing Better with Carrots

Nardia Boyer, a professional musician from Mountain View, California, writes:

I was startled by an improvement in vision after following the Eight-Week Program. In Week Two you suggested a carotene supplement. I peeled and juiced fresh carrots instead. Within one week a vision problem that had been plaguing me for three or four years cleared up. I was so astonished that I shared the good news with my ophthalmologist, who has since read your book.

This was the problem: I am a performing harpist, and I was seeing double strings after a short time playing, especially if the light was moderate. My first glasses were prescribed four years ago, when I was forty-six. This summer, as I played music for a wedding, I took off the glasses to see the minister and watch for cues. I glanced back at my music—it was perfectly clear! I was startled to be rid of this sight problem. I played the rest of the day *and* that evening, in moderate light, *with no glasses*. And have ever since.

7

WEEK THREE

Projects

• Find out where you can buy organic produce. Inquire in grocery stores or health-food stores, or use the resource guide in the appendix. Make a commitment to buy organically produced fruits and vegetables, especially the ones mentioned on page 84 as being the most likely to carry unhealthy residues of agrichemicals.
• If you use an electric blanket, stop. Remove electric clock radios from the immediate vicinity of your bed. If you use an older computer, buy a radiation shield for the video display of the monitor. Buy a pair of UV-protective sunglasses if you do not have any.

Diet

• Make a conscious effort to eat an extra serving of fruits and vegetables with at least one meal this week.
• Eat fish at least twice this week.
• Replace at least one serving of meat with a soy food of your choice.

Supplements

• With lunch or your largest meal take 400 to 800 IU of vitamin E and 200 to 300 micrograms of selenium.

Exercise

• Increase your daily walk to twenty minutes. If you do other aerobic exercise, consider cutting it back to two or three days, substituting an aerobic walk on the other days.
• Do some simple stretching to improve your flexibility (see pages 95–6 for examples).

Mental/Spiritual

• Add the next exercise to your breath work. This one is called "Letting Yourself Be Breathed," and you will find it described on pages 96–7.
• Ask friends and bookstore clerks about inspirational books they recommend. Make a list of some you would like to read in the areas of spirituality, self-help, poetry, biography, or any other category, and select one that you will begin this week.
• Make a list of friends and acquaintances in whose company you feel more alive, happier, and more optimistic. Resolve to spend some time with one of them this week.
• Remember to abstain from news again one day this week.

Optional (but Highly Recommended)

• Buy more flowers.
• Find out how to grow some of your own food, even if just in containers on a terrace or patio.

COMMENTARY

Projects

Both projects this week involve taking further steps to protect yourself from toxins: chemical toxins in food and energetic toxins in the home. Cumulative toxic damage is a chief reason for failure of the healing system as people age.

I cannot overemphasize the importance of becoming aware of toxic residues in food and working to reduce exposure to them. One reason for phasing out animal foods in your diet is to avoid the hormones and drugs they contain. Animals high on the food chain tend to concentrate environmental toxins, which accumulate, particularly, in fat. Shellfish are risky too because of their feeding habits and because we dump so much waste off our shores. Freshwater fish are hazardous because so much of the surface water all over the world is contaminated, and some ocean fish are definitely no longer safe, especially large, carnivorous fish like swordfish and marlin.

In the Eight-Week Program, you are going to be increasing your consumption of fruits and vegetables for their numerous health benefits. When it is ripe and good, fruit is a delight in the diet; it also provides vitamins, minerals, fiber, pigments with anticancer properties (I'm thinking of the red and purple proanthocyanidins in dark grapes and blueberries, for instance), and natural sugars that stress the pancreas much less than table sugar (sucrose). Vegetables are low in fat and calories, high in fiber, and full of health-protective factors.

But fruits and vegetables are often sprayed with pesticides, coated with fungicides, or full of toxins that were applied to the soil to be taken up by the roots of plants. One of the healthiest changes I see coming about in our society is the growth of organic agriculture in response to consumer demand for chemical-free produce. I encourage you to add your voice to the chorus making this demand. In some parts of the country, organic produce of excellent quality and variety is available at prices not much higher than those for regular produce. In other areas, it is unavailable, scarce, of uneven quality, and quite expensive. Depending on where you live, take advantage of the supply and buy organic as much as possible, or learn which crops are most likely to be contaminated and concentrate on finding organic versions of those. If you cannot, I recommend not eating them—at least not in quantity—or substituting other, safer foods.

A nonprofit research organization called the Environmental Working Group (see appendix for the address) reports periodically on health risks from pesticides in produce. The group says you can cut your exposure by 50 percent simply by reducing your consumption of the "dirty dozen"—the twelve fruits and vegetables they have found to be the most contaminated. At this writing, those twelve are strawberries, bell peppers (both green and red), spinach, cherries, peaches, Mexican cantaloupes, celery, apples, apricots, green beans, Chilean grapes, and cucumbers.

To this list, I would add wheat, soybeans, potatoes, and button mushrooms. By "wheat" I mean all products made from wheat and wheat flour: cereals, bread, crackers, cookies, and so forth. By "soybeans" I mean tofu, mock meats, and all other food items made from these versatile beans; since I want you to eat them, I urge you to look for organic brands. By "potatoes" I mean white (not sweet) potatoes. And by "mushrooms" I mean the common brown or white supermarket variety (*Agaricus brunnescens*).

In listing these foods, I am not exonerating other crops. I grow many of my own vegetables, but when my garden is not producing, I try to buy organic tomatoes, lettuce, broccoli. In southern Arizona, as in many other places, organic produce is not yet as abundant as it is in California, and it is often significantly more expensive than ordinary produce. It is worth knowing the crops that are most dangerous so you can prioritize your purchases or reduce consumption of those fruits and vegetables if you cannot find or afford organic versions.

I am well aware that many scientists and officials belittle concerns about chemical residues in our food, saying that the amounts present are too small to cause any harm. I see two fallacies in their argument. First, standards for acceptable levels of toxic agrichemicals in food are based on risks of acute toxicity—the possibility that exposure will cause immediate harm. They do not consider the risks of long-term cumulative damage to body defenses and healing ability. Second, those who argue that these chemical toxins are inconsequential to health fail to consider the possibility of synergy among them—that the effects of exposure to multiple toxins might together cause real harm.

An experiment reported in the June 7, 1996, issue of *Science* provides disturbing evidence for the latter possibility. A group of researchers from Tulane University used a novel system to assess the estrogenic effects of four pesticides: yeast cells genetically engineered to produce human estrogen. (See my commentary in chapter 6 about the estrogenic effects of pesticides and other environmental pollutants, which I believe to be factors in the worldwide epidemic of breast cancer.) The four chemicals tested on the yeast cells were all weakly estrogenic by themselves. But when two of them—endosulfan and dieldrin—were paired, the combined potency rose by factors of 160 to 1,600. In a news interview, the head of the research group said, "The thing that was most compelling was the dramatic synergy between two unlike chemicals. Instead of one plus one equaling two, we found that one plus one equals a thousand-fold. We expected interactions, but we were surprised they were so strong."

Endosulfan is one of the most widely used insecticides in the U.S., with about two million pounds applied annually on fruit, vegetable, and other crops. The EPA banned dieldrin in the 1980s, but it is a persistent contaminant in many parts of the country.

Protecting yourself from toxins is a crucial step in developing a healthy lifestyle. I have given you information about drinking water and what you can do to minimize health risks from it. Now I am telling you what you can do about food. Please take this advice seriously and act on it.

The kinds of toxins I have talked about so far are all material substances: heavy metals, agrichemicals, micro-organisms. I will now give you some suggestions for protecting yourself from toxic forms of energy. In some ways this is a harder subject to discuss, because some of the most dangerous forms of energy, like X-rays, are invisible or completely imperceptible. Also, medical science has paid little attention to the health hazards of electromagnetic pollution, and it is difficult to establish causal connections between exposure and diseases that might not show up until years later. Scientific evidence here is scant and contradictory, making the whole topic "controversial"; still, I think it would be foolish to take no action while waiting for the evidence to be uncovered.

I have written elsewhere about the hazards of ionizing radiation, the kind that is energetic enough to knock electrons out of their orbits and cause direct damage to DNA, increasing rates of mutation and cancer. X-rays and nuclear radiation are in this category. All that I will repeat here is a reminder that there is no such thing as a safe dose of radiation, since your risk of genetic and immune-system damage correlates with the total amount of radiation you have received over your lifetime, and any amount, however small, adds to that cumulative total and risk. *Never believe anyone who tells you that the amount of radiation coming at you from any source is too small to matter.*

In this section I am not going to be writing about ionizing radiation, which is now universally acknowledged to be hazardous to life. Rather, I am concerned about weaker forms of electromagnetic pollution that I believe pose subtler risks to our well-being and capacity for natural healing. You probably do not have X-ray machines or nu-clear waste around your home, but you very well might have appli-ances that generate electromagnetic fields. Even if the fields are weak, they may be able to disrupt the delicate biological mechanisms of the healing system, impairing its function over time and predisposing us to degenerative diseases as we age.

A most important fact about these environmental hazards is that the strength of the field falls off exponentially as distance increases between you and the source, so that putting even a little distance be-tween yourself and a source can give you great protection. For ex-ample, older computer monitors produce significant electromagnetic pollution (new models are well shielded), especially from the back of the monitor but also from the screen. You can buy shields that affix to the screen, but your best defense is to move yourself farther away.

I strongly recommend against using electric blankets and heating pads. They generate large electromagnetic fields and are used right next to the body. Use conventional blankets or down comforters on your bed, and if you need local heat, ask in drug- or medical-supply stores about nonelectric heating pads. I find them quite satisfactory. Another common household hazard is electric clock radios—the plug-in kind, not those that run on batteries. If you have one of these near your bed, do not keep it within a foot of your head. Also watch out for plug-in electric blow-driers for the hair; they are hazardous and, again, are used right near the brain.

On the other hand, I am not yet convinced of the dangers of cellu-lar telephones. So far, there is not enough information on their possi-ble biological effects. If you worry about them as a result of media reports suggesting an association with brain tumors, you can buy shielding sheaths that fit over the units.

Microwave ovens are another matter. Do not stand right next to them while they are operating, but, more important, use them only to defrost, reheat, or rapidly cook food. Long cooking of main dishes—say, for thirty minutes or more—can alter protein chemistry, creating new molecular species that might be harmful. Also, never microwave food in plastic containers or plastic wrap, because the microwave ra-diation can drive plastic molecules into the food; use only glass or ce-ramic containers, and waxed paper or a paper towel for a cover.

Speaking of microwaves, it is almost certainly dangerous to live in the proximity or path of microwave transmitters, such as those on military bases. (Another form of suspect radiation that is much used for long-distance military communications is ELF [extremely low-frequency] radiation.) It is also not a good idea to live under or next to power-transmission lines.

You will find more information about toxic forms of energy in the appendix.

Before I leave this subject, I must caution you about another source of unhealthy radiation that is totally familiar—the sun. Not only does it bathe our planet with vital heat and light, it also puts out a constant emission of ultraviolet (UV) and ionizing radiation. The earth's atmosphere filters out most of the most dangerous wavelengths, including nonsolar, cosmic radiation from outer space, but if you live at a high altitude, where there is less atmosphere above you, or spend a lot of time in airplanes, you will sustain significantly more exposure. And all of us on the surface of the earth are exposed to UV, more at some times of the day and year than at others.

UV is not ionizing, nor is it energetic enough to penetrate beneath the skin, but it can damage DNA in skin cells, causing mutations and malignant transformation. It is the primary cause of skin cancer, including the potentially deadly malignant melanoma, which is increasing at an alarming rate—the annual incidence has doubled since the 1980s. One reason for the change might be damage to the earth's ozone layer, which absorbs much of the ultraviolet radiation coming from the sun. Of course, UV also causes sunburn and premature aging of the skin and damages the eyes; in fact, it is a major cause of the two eye diseases responsible for most losses of vision in older people: cataracts and macular degeneration. The antioxidant formula you are learning to use in the Eight-Week Program helps your healing system defend the body against and repair UV damage, but it is not a substitute for knowing how to protect yourself from dangerous levels of exposure in the first place.

Two types of UV make their way through the atmosphere to your skin. UV-B rays cause sunburn and tanning (not a sign of health, but your skin's attempt to screen out the radiation) and until recently were thought to be the primary culprit in causing wrinkles, skin cancer, and other damage. Recent research shows, however, that UV-A rays, with longer wavelengths, may be even more of a problem, because they reach deeper into the skin, where they can damage underlying cells; it is UV-A that appears to promote melanoma. By the way, there are no "tanning" rays of the sun distinct from "burning" rays, despite propaganda to the contrary from the tanning-parlor industry. Tanning parlors are hazardous to health. Please stay out of them.

The first rule of sun protection is to stay out of the sun when the rays are strongest: from 10 a.m. to 2 p.m. standard time, within three months of the summer solstice, at low latitudes and high altitudes, and near reflective surfaces like water and white sand. A wide-brimmed hat can protect your face and neck from 70 percent of the sun's rays, but loose-meshed clothing is not much help. (A thin T-shirt has a sun-protective factor [SPF] of only 10.) Special sun-protective fabric with an SPF of 30 is now available—see the appendix for a source.

If you cannot stay out of the sun, I recommend using sunblock regularly, even getting in the habit of applying it to exposed areas of the body when you get up, as part of your morning ritual. Sunscreens were originally designed to block UV-B rays, but newer products block UV-A as well; check labels of products to be sure you get full protection. The SPF rating only reflects efficacy against UV-B and indicates how long you can stay in the sun without getting burned. Use a higher rather than a lower SPF product if you have a choice. Be sure to protect your children well and make them conscious of the danger; dermatologists say that even one severe sunburn in childhood significantly raises the risk of malignant melanoma in later life. Also watch for new sunscreen products that include antioxidant vitamins like C, E, and beta-carotene. These agents may boost the effectiveness of the screening agent and actually reduce the damage done by free radicals, the highly reactive molecules generated in the skin by UV.

Finally, always protect your eyes by wearing glasses that block UV, either sunglasses or ordinary glasses with a UV-blocking coating.

Diet

Here are vegetable recipes to try this week:

Vegetable Stocks

Vegetable dishes are greatly improved by using a vegetable stock instead of water. Here are three different versions of vegetable stocks for you to try. It is convenient to make them up and freeze them in batches for later use. If you have none on hand or do not have time to make your own stock, use instant vegetable broth powder from a natural-food store.

I

2 medium leeks
4 onions
6 carrots
3 stalks celery
1 small bunch parsley stems
1 tablespoon olive oil
2 teaspoons large-leaf marjoram
1/2 teaspoon dried thyme
3 Turkish bay leaves (or 1/2 California bay leaf)

1. Chop the leeks (which have been trimmed and well washed to remove any interior dirt; use white and light-green parts only), onions, carrots, celery, and parsley.
2. Heat the olive oil in a large pot, add the vegetables, and stir-fry to brown lightly. Add 1 1/2 gallons of cold water. Also add the marjoram, thyme, and bay leaves.
3. Bring to a boil, reduce heat, and simmer, partly covered, for 1 hour.
4. Strain stock through cheesecloth-lined strainer, cool, and chill or freeze.

II

1 large onion, chopped
1 large potato, unpeeled, cut into 1-inch chunks
2 leeks, prepared as in preceding recipe, sliced
2 large carrots, peeled and sliced
2 stalks celery, sliced
2 tomatoes, chopped
4 cloves garlic, chopped
1/4 cup chopped parsley
1 teaspoon dried basil

2 Turkish bay leaves
1/2 teaspoon dried thyme
1/4 teaspoon ground sage

1. Combine in a large pot: the onion, potato, leeks, carrots, celery, tomatoes, garlic, parsley, basil, bay leaves, thyme, sage, and 3 quarts of cold water.
2. Bring to a boil, reduce heat, cover, and simmer 1 hour.
3. Strain, cool, and chill or freeze.

III

6 large organic potatoes (see procedure below)
1 large onion, sliced
2 carrots, peeled and sliced
1 small stalk celery, sliced
sprig parsley
1 clove garlic, chopped

1. Wash the potatoes and remove the peels in strips at least 1/4 inch thick.
2. Place the peels in a large pot and use the potatoes in another recipe. To the pot add the onion, carrots, celery, parsley, and garlic.
3. Add 6 cups of cold water, bring to a boil, cover, reduce heat, and simmer slowly for 1 1/2 hours. Add water if necessary to keep the level constant.
4. Strain, cool, and chill, or freeze.

✌ *Barley and Vegetable Soup* ✌

3/4 cup medium pearl barley
11 cups vegetable stock (see preceding recipe)
2 tablespoons olive oil
1 1/2 cups chopped onion
1 cup chopped carrots
1/2 cup chopped celery
1 cup thinly sliced mushrooms

salt to taste
1/2 bunch parsley

1. In a saucepan, combine the barley and 3 cups of vegetable stock. Bring to a boil over medium heat, cover, and simmer for 1 hour, or until the liquid is absorbed.

2. Meanwhile, heat the olive oil in a large pot and add the onion, carrots, celery, and mushrooms. Cover and sweat the vegetables for about 5 minutes, until they begin to soften.

3. Add the remaining vegetable stock and simmer 30 minutes, covered.

4. Add the barley and simmer 5 minutes more. Add salt to taste and ladle into bowls. Serve garnished with some chopped fresh parsley.

⌘ *Braised Red Cabbage* ⌘

1 tablespoon olive oil
1 large onion, chopped
2 large carrots, peeled and sliced
1 large head red cabbage, cored and sliced 1/4 inch thick
1 large green apple, peeled, cored, and diced
salt to taste
3 large cloves garlic, mashed
1 Turkish bay leaf (or 1/3 California bay leaf)
1/4 teaspoon ground cloves
1 1/2 cups dry red wine
1/4 cup red wine vinegar
2 tablespoons light-brown sugar
1 cup peeled chestnuts (optional)

1. In a large pot, heat the olive oil. Add the onion and carrots and sauté over medium heat until onion is translucent.

2. Add the cabbage and apple and mix well, then add salt to taste, the garlic, the bay leaf, cloves, wine, vinegar, and sugar.

3. Bring to a low boil, cover, and cook for about 1 hour. Remove bay leaf and correct seasoning. (You may also add 1 cup of peeled chestnuts to cook in the braising liquid.)

✌ Roasted Root Vegetables ✌

*1–2 pounds root vegetables (use potatoes, carrots, parsnips, turnips,
rutabagas, beets), peeled and cut into 1-inch pieces
1 medium onion, peeled and cut into 1/4-inch wedges
2 tablespoons olive oil
salt to taste
1 head garlic, separated into cloves and peeled
herbs or balsamic vinegar (optional)*

1. Heat oven to 400°F. Place the root vegetables and the onion in a roasting pan.

2. Toss the vegetables with the olive oil and salt to taste. Do not crowd the vegetables.

3. Roast the mixture for 45–50 minutes, stirring every 15 minutes until they are tender and evenly browned. After half an hour, scatter the garlic cloves in with the vegetables.

4. Before serving, taste and add seasoning as you desire. You can sprinkle in fresh chopped herbs or add balsamic vinegar, for example.

✌ Grilled Vegetables ✌

*1 pound mixed vegetables (onions, mushrooms, red and green peppers,
carrots, sweet potatoes, eggplant), cut into bite-size chunks*

MARINADE
*1/4 cup olive oil
1/2 cup dry vermouth
1 tablespoon light-brown sugar
2 large cloves garlic, mashed
salt to taste
hot-pepper sauce (optional)*

ALTERNATE MARINADE
*1/4 cup natural soy sauce
1/2 cup sake or dry sherry
2 tablespoons light-brown sugar*

1 tablespoon dark-roasted sesame oil
2 teaspoons finely chopped fresh gingerroot

1. Prepare a charcoal or gas grill and lay out skewers.

2. Place the vegetables in a bowl and pour over them the marinade.

3. Marinate the vegetables for at least 15 minutes, then drain well and thread on skewers.

4. Grill the vegetables, turning skewers to achieve even cooking, until vegetables are tender and beginning to brown. Serve with rice.

Supplements

The vitamin E and selenium that you will start taking this week complete the antioxidant formula of the Eight-Week Program. Vitamin E is a powerful protector of the body; among its other properties, it blocks oxidation of LDL cholesterol, the kind that damages arteries but can only do so in oxidized form. It is not possible to get sufficient amounts of this vitamin from dietary sources, since it occurs mostly in oil-rich seeds. I recommend taking 400 IU a day if you are under age forty, 800 IU a day if you are forty or older. Be sure to take only natural vitamin E—the label will say "*d-* [not *dl-*] alpha-tocopherol with other tocopherols." If you cannot find the natural form in a drugstore, try a health-food store. There are newer, dry forms of vitamin E that come in tablets of 400 IU each; they may be more stable than oil-filled gel caps. Always take vitamin E with a meal to ensure proper absorption. I take mine with lunch.

Selenium is a trace mineral with proven cancer-fighting benefits. I recommend taking it together with vitamin E because the two enhance each other's absorption. (And I try not to take vitamin C at the same time, because C and some forms of selenium can interfere with each other's absorption.) I take 200 micrograms of selenium a day and recommend 300 micrograms as a daily dose for people who have had cancer or have increased risks of cancer for any reason.

Vitamin E is completely nontoxic. Selenium can be toxic in high doses—more than ten times the recommended amounts—but the first signs of overdose are easily noticeable—obvious peeling of fingernails and skin, and loss of hair.

Exercise

Stretching is the most natural form of nonaerobic exercise. I consider it an essential complement to aerobic conditioning and am introducing it this week as an ongoing part of the Eight-Week Program. You can learn a lot about our need to stretch by watching dogs and cats. They do it frequently, in various positions, especially on waking from sleep and after periods of activity. All of us tend to stretch after being in one position for a long time, and experts in human physiology say that we should develop habits of stretching in opposite ways from the positions we spend most time in during the day in order to condition our muscles and keep tendons, ligaments, and joints limber. For instance, if you work leaning over a desk, when you get home you should spend a few minutes with your head, neck, and shoulders arched backward.

Daily stretching is the best way to improve flexibility, one of the components of fitness. The more flexible your body is, the better it can meet the demands of life and resist injury. Besides, it just feels good to stretch. Animals look as if they are enjoying themselves when they do it; certainly dogs make sounds of pleasure as they stretch. Actually, the sensations of stretching often border on both pleasure and pain, but the end result is a welcome alteration of consciousness. Muscles contain stretch receptors, special groups of cells that inform the brain about their state of tension. This pathway of direct communication to the central nervous system probably explains why stretching can change our levels of arousal and moods so rapidly.

Stretching is so natural that you can easily invent your own forms of it. You will also find stretch classes at most fitness clubs, or can learn the techniques from books or videos (see the appendix for a source). I believe that, combined with the walking you will be doing in the Eight-Week Program, stretching will take care of most of the body's needs for physical conditioning. This week I want you to do five minutes of stretching every day. Do it when you come home from work, before you go to bed, or any other time you find convenient. Just do it.

Here are some examples of simple stretches to try. Avoid any tendency to hold your breath while doing them.

• Interlace your fingers, then straighten your arms out in front of you, palms facing out. Hold the stretch for twenty seconds, then rest for a few seconds and repeat it.
• Interlace your fingers, then turn palms upward above your head as you straighten your arms. Hold for ten seconds, rest, and repeat.
• Extend the arms to the side, palms facing forward, and stretch them backward. Hold for ten seconds, rest, and repeat.
• Hold your right arm just above the elbow with your left hand. Now gently pull your elbow toward your left shoulder while looking over your right shoulder. Hold for ten seconds. Repeat using the opposite arm and hand and looking over your left shoulder.
• Bend forward from a sitting position to stretch and relieve tension in the lower back. Hold for forty-five seconds, then put your hands on your thighs to help push your body back to an upright position.

You might also wish to explore yoga as as a formal system of stretching the body. Actually, this ancient Indian science is a philosophical-religious system for attaining unity of consciousness, but its physical component, known as *hatha yoga,* includes a number of *asanas,* or poses, which are what most people think of when they hear the word "yoga." You can learn these postures from books or videos, but it is easier to work with an instructor. Yoga classes are widely available through health clubs, community centers, and universities. You can practice on your own once you learn the basics, and need not spend a specified amount of time at it.

Looked at only as a very structured form of nonaerobic stretching, yoga offers several advantages. It tones all the muscles and balances all parts of the body, often dramatically increasing flexibility. (I recommend it for anyone suffering from chronic back pain.) It also produces deep relaxation and is a powerful stress-reducer. You can learn to do yoga at any age. Start out with beginning hatha yoga and do not attempt the very strenuous varieties (ashtanga, kundalini, Iyengar yoga, for example), which are beyond the scope of this Eight-Week Program.

Mental/Spiritual

The breathing exercise this week is a bit different, more of an exercise in imagination, and possibly more difficult. It takes little time, and if you succeed with it, I think you will find it unusually refreshing. I call it "Letting Yourself Be Breathed."

It is best done while lying on your back, so you might want to try it while falling asleep or on waking.

1. Close your eyes, letting your arms rest alongside your body, and focus attention on the breath without trying to influence it.

2. Now imagine that with each inhalation the universe is blowing breath into you and with each exhalation withdrawing it. Imagine yourself to be the passive recipient of breath. As the universe breathes into you, let yourself feel the breath penetrating to every part of your body, even to your fingers and toes.

3. Try to hold the perception for ten cycles of exhalation and inhalation. Do this once a day.

I've asked you also to think of friends and acquaintances who make you feel more alive, happy, and optimistic. Spend time with such people. Our spiritual selves resonate with others; if the interaction is positive, human connectedness is a most powerful healer, capable of neutralizing many harmful influences on the material plane.

Optional

Gardening is a healthy activity for many reasons. It connects you to nature, gives your body a workout, poses a variety of challenges that are satisfying to meet, and provides a chance to grow some of your own organic produce. Even if you live in an apartment, you can grow tomatoes, herbs, and flowers in window boxes and patio containers. You can also find out about participating in a community garden, which will give you a chance to join others in the effort.

A Healing Story:
Effects of Breathing Exercises

Mrs. F. E. of Ann Arbor, Michigan, writes:

I am a forty-three-year-old physical therapist who followed your Eight-Week Program. My objectives were to feel generally more healthy. I have struggled with chronic pain in my back and leg, as well as with minor depression. I have had various alternative treatments and was attracted to your plan because it integrated nutrition and mental/spiritual components nicely. (I had already begun several mental/spiritual interventions, which made following your plan easier.)

I think the breathing exercises were the most effective thing I added to my life. (I have since learned additional exercises from my reading.) I found deep relaxation as well as an increased ability to recall my dreams. Working with questions from a dream book, I have been able to sort out issues in my life much more quickly. This is enhanced by getting together regularly with friends who also write daily. These people have become my spiritual-growth friends.

It has been about ten months now since I started your plan, and I feel that the changes I've made are a permanent part of my life. I continue to integrate other strategies as well, and as a result of all the changes, I have to say that my health has improved even more. This fall was the first fall in fourteen years that I was free of an allergy to ragweed. My pain is much less, my energy is more even, and I have been able to be hopeful about complete health.

8

WEEK FOUR

Projects

• Check on your bed, mattress, and sleeping location. Is an uncomfortable bed or noisy bedroom interfering with restful sleep? Can you identify some other impediment to getting a good night's rest? If so, consider making the changes described on page 100.
• Find out about getting an air filter for your home or bedroom if you live in a polluted area or suffer from respiratory allergies, asthma, sinus problems, or other ailments that might be worsened by inhaled irritants.

Diet

• Eat some more garlic this week, in any form that appeals to you.
• Replace at least two meals of animal protein with soy protein.

Exercise

• Increase your aerobic walk to twenty-five minutes, five days of the week.

Mental/Spiritual

• Do two days of news fasting this week.

• Continue to practice the breathing exercises you have learned. This week you will add a powerful Relaxing Breath that will improve both mental and physical health (see page 108).

• Contact someone you know to have experienced healing or recovery from illness or injury. Ask for details of the experience.

Optional (but Highly Recommended)

• Try to observe a moment of gratitude for your food before meals, in any way that you find comfortable.

COMMENTARY

Projects

Adequate sleep is a key element of a healthy lifestyle; lack of it increases susceptibility to illness. I am sure you can look to your own experience to find instances when a good night's sleep nipped early illness in the bud and restored normal health. I know from my own experience that poor sleep is itself a sign of imperfect health and of a predisposition to further breakdown.

Common reasons for not sleeping well include a bed that is not right for you, a noisy bedroom, excessive stimulation from drugs or sensations during the day, bodily pain or discomfort, and mental or emotional disturbance—depression and anxiety, or an inability to stop thinking about bothersome events.

If you have any suspicion that your bed is not right for you, shop around for another one. Your mattress might be too soft or too firm, and your pillow might not be the right kind. You have many choices, from "orthopedic" mattresses to futons to air mattresses (including ones with dual controls, so that you and your sleeping partner can each get the degree of firmness that works best). Similarly, there is a wide choice of pillows, differing in shape and texture.

If your bedroom is noisy, the simplest solution is to buy a white-noise generator. I see these advertised in many mail-order catalogues and use one myself. They are inexpensive and effective, producing soothing sounds that mask jangling ones. Some have different settings to mimic ocean waves, waterfalls, or tropical rain.

Stimulant drugs, most often caffeine, are to blame for many cases of insomnia. Some people are so sensitive to the effect of caffeine on the sleep cycle that even one or two cups of a caffeinated beverage at breakfast will prevent them from falling asleep effortlessly many hours later. If you have problems falling asleep, pay attention to the amount of coffee, tea, cola, and chocolate you consume, and also check the caffeine content of any prescription and over-the-counter (OTC) drugs you may be taking. Also watch out for ephedra and ephedrine, the active components of many herbal diet and energy products sold in both drug- and health-food stores; pseudoephedrine, a decongestant in many OTC cold remedies; and phenylpropanolamine, found in OTC diet pills and cold remedies. All are strong stimulants that can interfere with sleep, depending on your sensitivity to them and the amounts you ingest.

If bodily pain or discomfort prevents you from getting good-quality sleep, it is especially important to pay attention to the design of your mattress. In addition, I recommend going to an osteopathic physician (D.O.) who specializes in OMT, osteopathic manipulative therapy (see appendix for information on how to locate one). A session or two of this safe and effective treatment can be life-changing.

If your mind is overactive, you will not be able to fall asleep even if you have the most comfortable bed and quietest bedroom in the world and never touch a drop of coffee or tea. Mental overactivity can also wake you after you have fallen asleep. It is very useful to learn to leave the day's worries behind when you get into bed. When my mind is very active, I often read until I drift off; a great many of the books I pick up—good or bad—are effective inducers of sleep. Also, I use the Relaxing Breath that I will teach you later in this chapter (see page 108). I cannot recommend it too highly as an aid to turning down the volume of thoughts and helping you fall asleep. Another possibility is to do a few stretches before you get into bed. Not only can this help balance your musculoskeletal system, it can also help you withdraw attention from thought by focusing it instead on the here and now of bodily sensations.

Doctors write innumerable prescriptions for hypnotic (sleep-inducing) drugs, and OTC sales of milder versions are also brisk. In my opinion, all of these sedatives are potentially dangerous, because of their addictiveness and their tendency to distort moods and compromise memory and intellectual function. A lesser-known hazard is that all sedatives suppress rapid-eye-movement (REM) sleep, the phase of sleep associated with dreaming that is necessary for good mental health. Do not rely on any of these drugs except for short-term management of situational insomnia—for example, because of a death in the family or loss of a job.

When I wrote *Spontaneous Healing,* the brain hormone melatonin had just come on the OTC market. It is a nontoxic regulator of the sleep-wake cycle that has become very popular despite warnings from neuroscientists who study it. I will repeat my opinion here that mela-tonin appears useful as a *short-term* strategy for managing jet lag and other disruptions of our biological clock but that I am very uneasy about people's taking it for more than a few nights in a row or over long periods of time. No one knows the full range of consequences of taking supplemental melatonin; in my view, there is reason to fear that it can disturb the delicate balance of our hormonal physiology and compromise health and healing in as-yet-unknown ways. If you want to try melatonin for international travel or situational insomnia, the best form to take is a sublingual (under-the-tongue) tablet that con-tains no more than 1 milligram of the hormone. (Break larger-dose forms in pieces.) Use it no more than one or two nights in a row to reset the sleep point of your internal clock, and do not use it at all if it causes nightmares or other untoward symptoms.

A much safer, natural sleep aid is the herb valerian, the root of a European plant, *Valeriana officinalis,* that human beings have used for centuries without indication of harm. You can buy tinctures of valerian root in health-food stores or pharmacies that stock natural products; the dose is 1 teaspoon in a little warm water at bedtime. Valerian is not addictive, but it is still a depressant and affects indi-viduals variably. Most people find it a very satisfactory hypnotic with no adverse effects. Some find it ineffective, a few become agitated on it, and a few report morning hangovers. I travel with a bottle of tinc-ture of valerian in case I need it, which I do only rarely. In any case, I do not recommend it for regular use or as a primary strategy for dealing with chronic insomnia.

I am also asking you this week to think about getting an air filter for your home, a protective strategy that is especially important if you suffer from respiratory disease of any sort, including allergies to inhaled irritants, but may be useful for anyone living in areas where the air is frequently dirty—the case for most urbanites, unfortunately. Two kinds of pollution make the air in many parts of the world a problem: particulate matter, including pollen, dust, and mold, and noxious gases from natural (volcanoes, forest fires) and human (automobiles, cigarettes, industry) activity.

Good technology now exists for removing particulate matter from the air inside your house in the form of high-efficiency particulate air (HEPA) filters that work very efficiently and are reasonably priced. You can buy free-standing models that will clear all particulate pollution from, say, your bedroom, or larger versions to be installed in the heating-and-cooling system of a whole house. I have seen many cases of dramatic improvement in respiratory health when patients followed this recommendation.

Gaseous pollution is harder to avoid and may be a chief reason for the increasing incidence of asthma, bronchitis, and sinusitis in the industrialized world, as well as a contributing factor to the development of lung cancer and emphysema. Some air-filtration systems include activated charcoal, which removes gaseous pollution as long as the charcoal is changed regularly. A simpler and greener strategy is to fill your home with house plants that are known to absorb toxic gases from the air. One of the most familiar is the spider plant (*Chlorophytum comosum*), which is very easy to grow, even tolerating low light. Other possibilities are Boston fern (*Nephrolepis exaltata bostoniensis*), English ivy (*Hedera helix*), and striped dracaena (*Dracaena marginata*).

If you are anxious about breathing polluted air, consider that the antioxidant formula you are taking will help your body neutralize the harmful effects of any toxins you do breathe in, that drinking plenty of pure water will help your body eliminate them, and that next week I'm going to explain why saunas and steam baths are another powerful way to strengthen your natural defenses against toxicity of all sorts.

Diet

I could—and probably will—write with passion about garlic (*Allium sativum*), one of my favorite flavors in cooking, whose health benefits have long been recognized in folk-medicine traditions around the world and now are increasingly, if grudgingly, acknowledged by medical researchers and practitioners. It is hard for me to imagine food prepared without garlic, and the smell of garlic cooking makes me feel immediately comfortable and at home in any kitchen or restaurant. I will also say right here and now that I have never minded the odor of garlic on anyone, and that one of the most obnoxious responses I get from radio and television hosts when I talk about the medicinal properties of this remarkable plant is, "Well, it will certainly keep everyone else away." If you eat garlic regularly—and others have a good attitude—any odor from it should hardly be noticeable.

Many scientific papers on garlic have appeared in recent years, and two international conferences have discussed its therapeutic properties. Above all, garlic is a superior tonic for the cardiovascular system. I will discuss tonics in detail in Week Six of this program. Here I will simply note that they are nontoxic, natural products that, if taken regularly over time, gradually tone or strengthen the body's innate systems of defense and healing. Typically, they have very general effects on more than one aspect of our physiology. For example, in addition to its wonderful influence on the heart and arteries, garlic is a powerful antibiotic and anticancer agent.

Garlic has three very important cardiovascular effects: One, it lowers blood pressure and is a key component in any natural approach to treating hypertension. Two, it lowers cholesterol and fats (triglycerides) in the blood, raising the protective (HDL) fraction of total cholesterol, while reducing the susceptibility of the harmful (LDL) fraction to oxidation and thereby diminishing its potential to damage artery walls. Three, garlic inhibits blood clotting by reducing the tendency of platelets to clump together. Platelet clumping on roughened walls of arteries damaged by atherosclerosis commonly initiates blood clots that lead to death of portions of the heart muscle (heart attacks). By all of these mechanisms, garlic offers protection against cardiovascular disease; epidemiologists think that high consumption of it in parts of Spain and Italy may contribute to a lower-than-expected incidence of coronary heart disease in those populations.

In addition, garlic is a strong antiseptic, counteracting the growth of many kinds of bacteria and fungi that can cause disease. It also boosts activity of the immune system, stimulating natural-killer (NK) cells, which are our main defense against cancer. Garlic appears to offer other protection from cancer as well, since it inactivates some of the carcinogens that people ingest and protects DNA from damage by others. As a natural antioxidant, garlic may also protect cells from degenerative changes, especially in the liver and brain.

To get all of these tonic effects, I suggest that you simply eat more fresh garlic in your food. Heat destroys some of the herb's properties, particularly the antibiotic ones, so add it near the end of cooking to preserve its benefits. If you can, eat a bit of raw garlic now and then: in very thin slices or minced fine, it is surprisingly good on sandwiches or in pasta or salads. (If this prescription is too strong for you, don't worry; just add more garlic to your cooking.) I'm not a fan of garlic powder or other dried and preserved forms, including the many brands of garlic pills on the market. The problem is that all of them are processed garlic that may or may not reproduce the many useful effects of the whole, fresh herb. The best of these products are standardized for content of allicin, the most studied of the family of sulfur-containing compounds in garlic, one that forms instantly when a garlic clove is cut, mashed, or otherwise exposed to air. But the chemistry of garlic is exceedingly rich, and I have not seen any evidence to convince me that allicin is the sole healthful component of garlic, or even the most important. I recommend against using garlic pills except as last resorts—if you are traveling, say, and simply can't get the real thing.

Here are this week's recipes, all featuring the real thing:

❧ *Garlic Broth* ❧

> *6 cups vegetable stock (see pages 89–91)*
> *1 1/2 tablespoons olive oil*
> *1/2 Turkish bay leaf*
> *1 head garlic, peeled and coarsely chopped*
> *1/4 teaspoon dried thyme*
> *pinch dried sage*
> *salt to taste*

1. To the vegetable stock add the olive oil, bay leaf, garlic, thyme, and sage.

2. Bring to a boil, reduce heat, cover, and simmer for 30 minutes. Add salt to taste.

3. Strain. Good as is, or use as a base for soups.

❧ Spinach with Garlic ❧

1 1/2 pound fresh spinach
2 teaspoons olive oil
1 head garlic, separated into cloves, peeled, and chopped
salt to taste
fresh lemon juice, balsamic vinegar, or red-pepper flakes (optional)

1. Wash the spinach well, drain, and remove large stems. If leaves are very large, cut them in half; otherwise leave them whole. Spinach cooks down to a surprising degree, so make sure you start with enough. One pound of fresh spinach will serve only 2–3 people as a side dish.

2. Heat the olive oil in a large, heavy skillet and add the garlic. Sauté, stirring, for 2 minutes.

3. Add the spinach in batches as it wilts down, and pour off any liquid that accumulates. Sauté just until all the spinach is wilted and bright green. Add salt if desired.

4. Serve as is or seasoned with one of the following: fresh lemon juice, balsamic vinegar, or red-pepper flakes.

❧ Bean Dip with Garlic ❧

1 jar bean dip
1 or 2 cloves garlic

1. Mash 1 or 2 cloves garlic into your favorite bean dip (there are some very good ones without added fat, both mild and spicy), mix well, and let sit at least an hour before serving.

❧ Pasta with Garlic and Oil ❧

This is an Italian classic, revised to give you more of the health benefits of the garlic by cooking it less.

1 pound dried pasta
1/4 cup olive oil

5 large cloves garlic, minced
salt to taste
hot red-pepper flakes or chopped fresh parsley (optional)

1. While the pasta is cooking, heat the olive oil in a small skillet and add the garlic cloves. Sauté for 1 minute.

2. Pour the mixture over the cooked, drained pasta and combine well. Season to taste with salt. Optional: consider sprinkling with hot red-pepper flakes or chopped fresh parsley.

✄ *Pasta with Garlic and Herbs* ✄

1 pound dried pasta
2 tablespoons olive oil
1 medium onion, diced
3 cloves garlic, minced
1 cup dry vermouth
salt to taste
1/4 teaspoon hot red-pepper flakes
1 teaspoon dried whole oregano
2 tablespoons chopped fresh basil (or 1 tablespoon dried basil)
1/4 cup chopped fresh parsley
grated Parmesan cheese (optional)

1. While the pasta is cooking, heat the olive oil in a skillet, add the onion, and sauté until it is translucent. Then add the garlic and sauté for a minute more.

2. Add the vermouth, salt to taste, the red-pepper flakes, oregano, basil, and parsley. Mix well and cook over medium-high heat for 5 minutes.

3. Pour over cooked, drained pasta, toss well, and serve with grated Parmesan cheese if desired.

Mental/Spiritual

You have two new tasks in this department this week: learn a new breathing exercise, the most important one of all, and interview someone about an experience of healing.

The breathing technique is an ancient one from the yogic tradition that I have written about in previous books, practice myself at least twice a day, and recommend to most patients who consult me. Here it is:

Place your tongue in the yogic position: touch the tip of your tongue to the inner surface of the upper front teeth, then slide it just above your teeth until it rests on the alveolar ridge, the soft tissue between the teeth and the roof of the mouth. Keep it there during the whole exercise. Now exhale completely through the mouth, making an audible sound (a *whoosh*). Then close your mouth and inhale quietly through your nose to a (silent) count of four. Then hold your breath for a count of seven. Finally, exhale audibly through the mouth to a count of eight. This constitutes one breath cycle. Repeat for a total of four cycles, then breathe normally. If you have difficulty exhaling with your tongue in place, try pursing your lips; you will soon get the knack of how to do it. Note that the speed with which you do the exercise is unimportant. What is important is the ratio of four, seven, eight for inhalation, hold, exhalation. You will be limited by how long you can comfortably hold your breath, so adjust your counting accordingly. As you practice this exercise, you will be able to slow it down, which is desirable. Do it at least twice a day.

You can practice this Relaxing Breath anywhere, but if you are seated, try to keep your back straight. I do it in the morning, before I meditate, and in the evening, when I am lying in bed, just before going to sleep. It helps me fall back to sleep if I happen to wake during the night, and it also helps me disengage from thought and calm emotional upset. I think of it as a kind of tonic, a spiritual rather than a material one, with wonderful effects on the involuntary nervous system. Specifically, it increases the ratio of parasympathetic to sympathetic nervous-system activity, decreasing internalized anxiety and yielding more harmonious functioning of the digestive, circulatory, and other systems. The benefits are gradual and cumulative, leading eventually to better health of the whole nervous system. It is also a specific treatment for high blood pressure, cold hands, irritable bowel syndrome, benign cardiac arrhythmias, anxiety disorder and panic disorder, and a variety of other common ailments. Above all, it is the most effective and time-efficient relaxation method I have found. Please work with it conscientiously.

In Week One of this Eight-Week Program I asked you to think of your own experiences of healing. Now I am asking you to inquire among people you know to try to learn about a healing experience in a more formal way. As you know, collecting such stories is a main interest of mine, and as I've written and spoken more on the subject, they come to me more frequently. I think it is vitally important to get these accounts increasingly circulated, to re-establish the concept of spontaneous healing at the center of our thinking about health and illness. The most limiting omission in conventional medicine today is the absence of the concept that the body can repair itself. Not only does it represent a marked deviation from Western medicine of the past and from the traditions of other therapeutic systems, like those from China and India, it is also responsible for the great emphasis on intervention in contemporary medicine, particularly with methods that rely heavily on technology and, as a result, are expensive and invasive and often produce harm.

One of my missions is to get people thinking about healing, talking about it, investigating it. A good place to begin is with your own circle of relatives, friends, and associates. You do not have to go looking for a case of cancer remission. Less dramatic kinds of healing are equally interesting, whether from injury, acute or chronic illness, or, really, any ailment. Ask for details. What did the person do, in his or her own mind, that allowed the healing system to take care of the problem? Did he or she use treatment? Did the experience change ways of thinking about the body and about dealing with illness in the future?

The more you bring the concept of healing into everyday awareness, the greater will be your confidence in your inborn ability to deal with lapses in health, both minor and major, common and uncommon.

Optional (but Highly Recommended)

The point of bringing a spiritual perspective into your life is to remind yourself that you are more than just your physical body, that there is more to life than the material universe.

We are spiritual beings inhabiting material forms, but the immediacy and substantiality of matter make it very easy to fall into the delusion that nothing exists beyond what we perceive with the five senses. Logic should help us out of that delusion, since it is clear that what we perceive is a narrow slice of the whole. Consider vision, for example: our eyes can only see a small portion of the electromagnetic spectrum. What would things look like if we could see infrared and ultraviolet as well? What would it be like to have the olfactory awareness of a dog, the auditory ability of a bat, the tactile sensitivity of a snake? Surely the horizons of our reality would expand, though we might still think there was nothing beyond our extended world of the senses.

In fact, logic is not a very useful tool to deal with the delusion that our senses define the limits of reality. Instead, it seems necessary to make ourselves remember, again and again, at every possible opportunity, that we are more than physical bodies, that there is more to life than material existence. A good time for doing this is when we sit down to eat. Most of us eat three times a day or more, so there is no shortage of opportunity. Moreover, the act of eating offers a profound glimpse into the mystery of life and the strange interconnectedness of spirit and matter. Life lives at the expense of other life. It matters not whether you are a carnivore or a vegetarian; you perpetuate your material existence by depriving other organisms of theirs. The recycling of forms in this way is a useful focus for contemplation, and we have a chance to look at it squarely every time we eat. I find it a useful technique for raising spiritual awareness to take a moment before eating to remember our dependence on other living things and our need to take life in order to sustain life. I do not want to impose any particular form or ritual on you, only to urge you to take advantage of this opportunity that comes around so often to remind yourself of your essential nature and relationship to the universe. You may already be in the habit of saying some sort of grace aloud or to yourself, which is fine. Or you may simply want to take a moment, however brief, to feel gratitude for the food you are about to eat. Or you may just want to close your eyes and focus on your breath for a moment before you dig in. Experiment. If you can find a practice that works for you, you will develop a habit that can be very useful in moving you away from delusion and toward reality. Ancient Eastern thinkers tell us this is the direction in which we will find freedom and comfort. Enough said.

A HEALING STORY:
GIVING THE LIVER A CHANCE

FREYA DIAMOND of Santa Fe, New Mexico, is in good health at age fifty-two. She is also a solid proponent of natural medicine. But when I first met her as a patient in 1986, she was in turmoil, having just learned she had a serious illness, one with a grim prognosis. Here is the story in her own words, with my comments in brackets:

When I saw you, I had just been diagnosed with chronic, active hepatitis by two prominent gastroenterologists in Los Angeles. The diagnosis was indicated by extensive blood tests and confirmed by liver biopsy. These doctors, who were the best in the area, could not determine the cause but thought it was an autoimmune process, not an infection, and told me I had to take immunosuppressive drugs. I received prescriptions for prednisone and Imuran [azathioprine, a drug often given to organ-transplant recipients to prevent rejection, one that is mutagenic, carcinogenic, and distributed with a long list of warnings about its toxicity]. My doctor told me I would most likely have to take them indefinitely. I had previously taken prednisone for Crohn's disease and was aware of its many side effects. Frankly, I was terrified of going on these drugs and getting back on the medical merry-go-round, but both doctors warned me that not doing so would surely result in terrible illness and a shortened life. I also hesitated because I did not feel as sick as the doctor said I was.

Fortunately, I was able to meet with you, after a mutual friend encouraged me to seek out alternative approaches to treatment. You told me about the great regenerative power of the liver and recommended a vitamin regimen [the antioxidant formula of the Eight-Week Program], milk-thistle seed [an herbal remedy, *Silybum marianum,* that is nontoxic and protects liver cells from injury], a low-protein diet, and relaxation techniques—all of which I followed. In addition, you suggested I try to find a local physician who would be willing to monitor my liver function and not insist on the use of immunosuppressive drugs, one with an open mind to the course I wanted to follow to heal myself.

Within several months, all my liver-function tests were normal. The gastroenterologist I selected was both pleased and astonished, as was I. It has now been ten years, and aside from one short period, I have had totally normal blood tests and been completely symptom-free. That one period of abnormality coincided with my going back briefly on an antibiotic, Minocin, that I had been taking for acne off and on for years when I received the initial diagnosis. [Minocin is a semisynthetic derivative of tetracycline often given long-term for the treatment of acne; along with more common adverse reactions, it has, in rare instances, caused elevated levels of liver enzymes, hepatitis, and liver failure.] I had stopped taking it along with all other medication when my liver problem was diagnosed, and I now believe, as does the gastroenterologist, that the Minocin had a lot to do with the original diagnosis. If it weren't for the alternatives that you recommended and I chose to follow, I would be on other powerful and toxic drugs for the rest of my life, believing they were necessary for my continued good health.

That series of events has completely changed the way I view standard medicine and the alternative possibilities that exist for health and healing.

9

WEEK FIVE

Projects

• Locate a steam bath or sauna that you can use. Use it for up to twenty minutes one day. It should be hot enough to make you sweat freely; be sure to drink plenty of pure water to replace lost fluid.

Diet

• Buy a piece of fresh gingerroot and make yourself some ginger tea, as described on page 119. Also try some crystallized ginger to see if you like it.

Exercise

• Increase your aerobic walk to thirty minutes, five days of the week.

Mental/Spiritual

• Extend your news fast to three days this week.
• Practice daily the breathing exercises you have learned, and add the Stimulating Breath procedure described on page 122.
• Listen to a piece of music that you find inspirational and uplifting.
• Bring more flowers into your home this week.

Optional

• Try a one-day "fruit fast," eating as much fresh fruit as you like but nothing else except water and herbal tea. Take vitamin C but skip the other supplements on this day.

COMMENTARY

You have reached a milestone in the Eight-Week Program: the halfway point. By now you have made significant changes in your diet, your physical activity, and your breathing. You have started protecting your healing system by consuming particular foods and supplements, and you have been improving mental and spiritual health as well. In the coming month, you will be consolidating these changes, refining them, and adding other elements to your new, healthier lifestyle. Remember that you should be following all the recommendations of previous weeks, adding this week's steps to your developing program.

Projects

Let me talk to you first this week about the value of sweating. In addition to its well-known function of cooling the body by evaporation in hot weather, it is one of our most important mechanisms of natural healing, since it allows the body to rid itself of unwanted materials. If you eat too much sodium, you can eliminate the excess in sweat. The body can also eliminate other minerals, drugs, and some toxins by this route, taking part of the workload off the liver and kidneys, which are chiefly responsible for detoxification and purification of the blood. (That is why I recommend regular sweating to anyone with liver or kidney disease.)

In many cultures, sweat bathing is an important ritual, used for both hygienic and spiritual ends. The Native American sweat lodge, which I have written about elsewhere, is a well-known example, with a distinctly spiritual emphasis. It is becoming more and more popular throughout the world with the revival of Lakota religion and its vigorous diffusion far beyond the homelands of that remarkable people. To most Americans, who regard sweat bathing as a purely secular activity, the idea of praying while sweating or feeling closer to the

Great Spirit as a result will seem strange, but the fact is that people throughout history have been fascinated with the concepts of pollution and purification and have regarded purification of the body to be inseparable from purification of spirit. Of course, the Native American ideal of medicine embraces not only our concept of medicine, directed at the physical body, but also religion and magic. It has always seemed to me that we could do well by similarly enlarging our vision of medicine.

Even in Finland, which gave us the sauna, the practice, although often appearing social and secular, has deeper associations, as spelled out in *The Sauna Book* by Tom Johnson and Tim Miller:

> For the Finns "sauna" is a concept infused with a special mystique, an ideal, transcending the grubbiness of day-to-day activities. So reverent are the Finns toward sauna that they rank it in holiness with the church. This esteem is drawn from ancient traditions; one is the belief that fire is holy, an object of worship, and in such a belief system the sauna stove easily becomes transformed into an altar.

In asking you to take up the practice of sweat bathing, I cannot separate its physical and spiritual aspects. Sweating is clearly good for the bodies of most people; in my experience, it is also highly salutory for our minds and spirits.

You can sweat in dry heat or wet heat or a combination of the two. Many people think of a sauna as a wood-paneled room with an electrically heated stove that maintains an air temperature of 160° to 210°F. (71° to 98°C.) and humidity at a low 10 percent, but in the authentic Finnish version, a wood fire is used to heat a stove piled with rocks that can be doused with water to create steam, easily raising the humidity to 30 percent. Finns like cycles of dry and wet heat, always followed by a plunge into cold water. You can take much higher temperatures of dry heat than wet heat, because steam conducts heat to your body more efficiently than air. A steam room feels very hot at 115°F. (47°C.).

Whether you prefer dry or wet heat may depend in part on how much you sweat. Sweating is one way that the body can dissipate heat; the lower the humidity, the better it works. Women have a lower density of sweat glands in the skin than men, but there is much individual variation in this characteristic. If you are a less copious sweater, you might do better in drier heat. I find the purely dry air of an electric sauna irritating to my nasal passages and my respiratory system and like to be able to create some steam. I also like steam rooms very much, enjoying the noise of steam coming out of vents and the dreamy, visual quality of the resulting fog. And I am a copious sweater. You will have to experiment to find what suits you best.

People easily learn to acclimate to sweat bathing, to take hotter and hotter temperatures for longer periods. If you have never done it before, start gently and increase exposure gradually. Although it may feel as if you are baking or boiling, your core temperature rises only slightly in a steam or sauna; it is surface temperature that goes up significantly. Sweat bathing induces dramatic changes in physiology, especially in cardiovascular function, but recovery is rapid once you leave the hot chamber, and *unless you have significant cardiovascular disease,* the changes probably give the heart and arteries a healthy workout.

Medical opinion is divided on the benefits and hazards of sweat bathing, but I find the differences often to be culturally based. Finnish scientists generally minimize the risks of sauna, and Finnish doctors commonly recommend it for pregnant women up to the day of delivery. American doctors shudder at that prescription, generally warning patients away from steam rooms and saunas. (No doubt you have seen the cautionary signs that health clubs feel obligated to post on the doors of these facilities.) Having watched very sick people emerge from scalding Indian sweat lodges not only unharmed but actually much improved, I am inclined to regard most of the medical caution as unfounded. I frequently recommend regular sweat bathing to patients with a variety of ailments, from infectious disease to arthritis and drug addiction, and find it to be a most useful addition to a natural treatment regimen. Nevertheless, check with your physician if you have high blood pressure, heart disease, or other ailments before you follow my recommendation for sweating.

Try to locate a convenient sauna or steam room this week and take a good sweat bath one day. Be sure that you are well hydrated before you enter, and be sure to drink enough water when you finish to replace what you lose. If you can finish with a cold plunge or shower, try that too. Many people find that it leaves them glowing with vitality. Note the effects of the sweat bath on your energy level, mood, state of tension, and sleep, as well as any effects on your skin, muscles, and joints.

Diet

Your dietary prescription this week is to get to know more about ginger. Ginger is the underground stem (rhizome) of a plant, *Zingiber officinale,* native to tropical Asia. The designation *officinale* represents the plant's official status in medicine of the past. From ancient times, doctors in both China and India regarded ginger as a superior medicine, adding it to combination remedies for its tonifying and spiritually uplifting properties. People throughout the world have learned to value its warming effect and ability to stimulate digestion, settle upset stomachs, and relieve aches and pains. A very popular folk remedy in Japan is the ginger compress: grated fresh ginger is mixed with a little hot water, spread on a clean cloth, and applied to any part of the body that is sick or hurting. It is covered with hot cloths and changed frequently. This method is said to draw toxins, infection, and even malignant growth to the surface of the body, where it can be discharged.

In recent years, a great deal of medical research, much of it in Japan and Europe, has documented remarkable therapeutic effects of ginger and its components. American doctors tend to be unaware of these studies. The chemistry of ginger is complex, with more than four hundred compounds known to contribute to the plant's fragrance, taste, and biological activity. Much of the focus of research has been on two groups of these that account for ginger's pungency: the gingerols and the shogaols (*shoga* is the Japanese name for ginger). In addition, the rhizome contains enzymes and antioxidants that are probably also key components.

The tonic effects of ginger on the digestive system are clear: it improves the digestion of proteins, is an effective treatment for nausea and motion sickness, strengthens the mucosal lining of the upper GI tract in a way that protects against the formation of ulcers, and has a wide range of actions against intestinal parasites. Chinese cooks use fresh ginger in most dishes in part because they believe it neutralizes the undesirable qualities of other ingredients, especially fish and meat, that might produce indigestion.

Other well-studied actions of ginger affect the synthesis and deployment of a group of biological response moderators called *eicosanoids,* which mediate healing and immunity. The body makes these important compounds from essential fatty acids and uses them to regulate critical cellular functions. Three principal categories of eicosanoids—prostaglandins, thromboxanes, and leukotrienes—are much in the medical news as subjects of ongoing research. Imbalances in eicosanoid synthesis and release underlie many common illnesses, from arthritis and peptic ulcer to the increased platelet aggregation that can trigger heart attacks and strokes. Ginger modulates this system in ways that reduce abnormal inflammation and clotting. It may be as effective as some of the nonsteroidal anti-inflammatory drugs that are now in such widespread use, but much less toxic, because it protects the lining of the stomach instead of damaging it. It is as a modulator of eicosanoids that ginger may be most helpful to the healing system.

Additionally, ginger tones the circulatory system and has anti-cancer effects, blocking the ability of some carcinogens to cause mutations in DNA.

You can take ginger in the form of the fresh rhizome (peeled, grated, and finely chopped or squeezed for its juice) or as candied slices (crystallized ginger), honey-based syrups, or encapsulated extracts. At the end of this section, I will tell you how to prepare fresh gingerroot tea, a delightful and healthful beverage, and I will give you a number of recipes for favorite dishes that feature this strong-flavored plant. I happen to like crystallized ginger and use it to satisfy my sweet tooth as well as give my taste buds a zing. If you find it too pungent to eat that way, try nibbling small bits with raw almonds or dried fruit. I'd like you to experiment with ways of adding ginger to your diet on a regular basis, since I consider it a generally useful tonic.

When ginger is dried, its chemistry changes; in particular, the gingerols, which are abundant in the fresh rhizome, convert to the more pungent shogaols. These two classes of compounds have different properties, with shogaols having more powerful anti-inflammatory and analgesic effects. Therefore, it might be wise to use more than one form of ginger, and persons with arthritis or other inflammatory conditions might get more benefit from capsules of dried, powdered ginger, which are available in health-food stores. Typical capsules contain 500 milligrams of the spice, and a usual dose is 1 to 2 grams a day. Start with one capsule twice a day with meals. Ginger is nontoxic, but if you take the powdered form on an empty stomach, you might experience heartburn.

Here are some recipes featuring ginger:

⁓ *Ginger Tea* ⁓

In this recipe, gingerroot should be peeled and grated lengthwise on the large holes of a grater.

1/2 teaspoon grated fresh gingerroot (see headnote)
1/2 teaspoon honey, or to taste

1. For an individual serving, put the ginger into a cup of boiling water, cover, and let it steep for 10–15 minutes.
2. Strain, add honey to taste, and drink hot or iced.

You can also buy honey-based ginger syrups in health-food stores and add them to hot, cold, or sparkling water for an instant beverage. Or you can make your own ginger syrup by adding one part of grated fresh ginger to three parts of raw, mild-flavored honey; keep this in the refrigerator.

⁓ *Ginger-Carrot Soup* ⁓

3 cups carrots
1 medium potato
8 cups vegetable stock (see pages 89–91)
1 medium onion
2 teaspoons canola oil
3 tablespoons finely chopped fresh gingerroot
salt to taste
dash of dry sherry
dash of nutmeg
chopped fresh parsley or cilantro (optional)

1. Peel and slice the carrots and potato and put in a pot with the vegetable stock.
2. Bring to a boil, cover, reduce heat, and boil gently until the vegetables are tender, about 30–45 minutes.
3. Meanwhile, chop the onion.
4. Heat the canola oil in a skillet, add the onion and ginger, and sauté, stirring, just until onion is translucent. Remove from heat.

5. When carrots and potato are tender, add the onion and ginger to the pot, and cook together for 5 minutes.

6. Puree the soup in batches in a blender or food processor. Add salt to taste and flavor with the sherry and nutmeg. Serve plain or garnished with chopped fresh parsley or cilantro.

ᴥ Chinese Green Bean Salad ᴥ

1 pound fresh organic green beans
1 tablespoon finely chopped fresh gingerroot

DRESSING
4 teaspoons dry mustard powder
1 tablespoon cold water
2 teaspoons sugar
2 tablespoons reduced-sodium soy sauce
3 tablespoons rice or cider vinegar
2 teaspoons dark-roasted sesame oil

1. Trim and slice the beans crosswise, into 1-inch lengths. Cook in rapidly boiling water about 5 minutes, or until crunchy-tender.

2. Drain beans, chill in cold water, and drain well. Toss with the gingerroot and the dressing. Mix the dressing before tossing it with the beans.

ᴥ Stir-Fried Bean Sprouts ᴥ

1 pound fresh mung-bean sprouts
1 tablespoon canola oil
3 scallions, split lengthwise and cut into 1-inch strips
1 tablespoon finely chopped fresh gingerroot
1/2 teaspoon light-brown sugar
salt to taste
red-pepper flakes, natural soy sauce, or rice vinegar (optional)

1. Wash and drain the bean sprouts.

2. Heat the canola oil in a wok or skillet, add the scallions and ginger, and stir-fry over high heat for a few seconds. Then add the

bean sprouts and stir-fry for 1 minute. Do not overcook; sprouts should remain crunchy but lose their raw bean taste.

3. Add the brown sugar and salt to taste. Mix well and serve. Optional: add pinches of red-pepper flakes or dashes of natural soy sauce and rice vinegar.

❧ *Fruit Salad with Crystallized Ginger* ❧

3 cups sliced fresh fruit
3 slices crystallized ginger, minced finely
1 cup freshly squeezed orange juice

1. Add crystallized ginger to the fruit.
2. Pour a cup of orange juice over the fruit, mix well, and let sit for at least 30 minutes before serving.

❧ *Ginger-Almond Pears* ❧

5 firm, ripe pears
3 cups apple cider
2 teaspoons finely chopped fresh gingerroot
salt to taste
3 tablespoons arrowroot starch
1/2 teaspoon pure almond extract

1. Peel the pears, quarter them lengthwise, and core. Slice pears thinly and place in a saucepan with the apple cider and gingerroot. Add a pinch of salt.
2. Bring to a boil, reduce heat, and simmer until pears are tender, about 15 minutes.
3. Dissolve arrowroot starch in 1/3 cup cold water and add to the simmering pears, stirring, until the sauce is thick and clear.
4. Remove from heat and stir in almond extract. Serve warm or cold.

Mental/Spiritual

Here is a new breathing exercise to try this week, also from the tradition of yoga. It is stimulating rather than relaxing, and therefore you can use it to wake yourself up if you are feeling drowsy or mentally sluggish.

1. Sit comfortably with your back straight, eyes closed, and your tongue in the yogic position, as you learned for the Relaxing Breath last week. Keep it there during the whole exercise.
2. Breathe in and out rapidly through the nose, keeping your mouth lightly closed. Inhalation and exhalation should be equal and short, and you should feel muscular effort at the base of the neck just above the collarbones and at the diaphragm. (Try putting your hands on these spots to get a sense of the movement.) The action of the chest should be rapid and mechanical, like a bellows pumping air; in fact, the Sanskrit name for this exercise means "bellows breath." Breath should be audible on both inhalation and exhalation, as rapid as three cycles per second if you can do that comfortably.

The first time you try this exercise, do it for just fifteen seconds, then breathe normally. Each time you do it, increase the duration by five seconds, until you get up to a full minute. This is real exercise, and you can expect to feel fatigue of the muscles you are using. (Of course, they will become stronger with practice.) You will also begin to feel something else: a subtle but definite movement of energy through the body when you return to normal breathing. I feel it as a vibration or tingling, especially in my arms, along with greater alertness and dissipation of fatigue. This is not hyperventilation (which produces physiological changes as a result of blowing off excess carbon dioxide) but a way of activating the central nervous system. Once you can do the bellows breath for a full minute, try using it instead of caffeine as a pick-me-up in the afternoon. I find it particularly useful if I start to feel sleepy while driving. You can also use this exercise to warm yourself up if you are feeling cold. The more you use it, the more you will become aware of the energy it creates.

This completes the set of five breathing techniques that are an essential component of this Eight-Week Program. Let me review them for you and suggest how you might use them in your daily routine from now on.

Breath Observation, which you learned in Week One, is a meditation practice that will help you relax, and will be a great asset to you if you get in the habit of doing it regularly. I have asked you to do it for five minutes a day throughout this program, but you are welcome to extend that time as much as you want. I find that, if I do not meditate in the morning, before I get caught up in the day's activities, I tend not to do it at all; by bedtime I am usually too tired to make myself do it. Therefore, I recommend taking five minutes in the morning for this practice. At the end of the program, if you increase the time, you can experiment with ways of fitting it in to your schedule.

The mental Reversal of Inhalation and Exhalation that you learned in Week Two will help you develop your breathing capacity and thereby improve your health in general. I have asked you to do it for a minute a day, but you can also do it whenever you remember to, whenever you have an idle moment. One possibility is to tack it onto the five-minute period of Breath Observation.

The imaginative play that I call Letting Yourself Be Breathed, which I taught you in Week Three and asked you to do once a day for ten breath cycles, can also be done anywhere and anytime, but you may find it easiest to do lying down, when you get into bed at night or when you first wake up in the morning.

The formal Relaxing Breath that you learned last week requires at least two sessions of four breath cycles each. When you finish the program, I will ask you to increase this to eight cycles twice a day. Of course, you can also do this exercise anytime that you feel anxious, upset, or in physical discomfort of any sort, and I encourage you to do so, but two sessions are mandatory. I like to do one of them in the morning before I meditate, because it naturally puts me in a meditative state. I do the other in bed at night, just before falling asleep.

Finally, the Stimulating Breath that you just learned is suitable for use anytime, once you get up to speed with it for a full minute. As I told you, it is very useful for waking yourself up if you feel drowsy or mentally cloudy, but I want you to practice it at least once a day, no matter what. I find that doing it just before the Relaxing Breath further enhances a meditative state, so I incorporate it in my morning ritual.

Here, then, is one possibility for arranging the five breathing exercises of this program:

Morning: Stimulating Breath, followed immediately by
               Relaxing Breath, followed immediately by
               Breath Observation (minimum five minutes), followed immediately by
               Reversal of Inhalation and Exhalation
Bedtime: Let Yourself Be Breathed (ten breaths), followed immediately by
               Relaxing Breath

All of this takes less than ten minutes and can bring you remarkable improvements in health. I think you will enjoy this assignment, and I think you will find that you will drift off to sleep quite pleasantly after the evening session. Remember that the benefits of breath work depend on daily practice and develop gradually and cumulatively.

In addition to the usual recommendations to bring flowers into your home, I've asked you to think of a piece of music you find inspirational and uplifting and to listen to it. Music has a special power to influence consciousness. It is often the sound track of a scary movie, more than the images on the screen, that gives people goosebumps and chills. Many cultures around the world recognize this power of music. Some forbid it (Islamic fundamentalists), others use it in rituals designed to alter consciousness (voodooists). The essential tool of the shaman is a drum. By using particular rhythms, he or she can leave the physical body and journey to the spirit realm. Once, I had the pleasure of listening to a large gamelan ensemble play in Chicago's Field Museum. Gamelan is the traditional music of Bali, produced by a variety of gongs and percussion instruments. One piece I heard—and felt—that night was a traditional composition used to rouse warriors before battle. By the end of it, I was feeling powerful adrenaline surges throughout my body and was ready to smash something. In African religion, drumming is a highly developed art, capable of inducing spectacular changes in awareness, including sexual excitement, trance, spirit possession, and even complete loss of consciousness.

One of the highest purposes of music is to raise spiritual energy and put us more in touch with the higher self. I would not presume to recommend particular compositions or even types of music to you, because musical preference is strongly culturally conditioned and a matter of individual taste. As with food, one person's meat (or, better, salmon) is another's poison. Handel's "Hallelujah Chorus" certainly pleases me, but so does Creedence Clearwater Revival's "Lookin' Out My Back Door." If the musical key to your higher self is "Home on the Range" or the "Marine Hymn," that's your business—go for it! Just make a point of listening to it this week and, perhaps, preparing a list of other musical compositions that also uplift your spirits. Try to bring these experiences into your life on a regular basis, throughout the remaining weeks of this program and after you complete it.

Optional

If you are inclined to experiment, I would like you to consider a "fruit fast" this week. I put that phrase in quotation marks because a fast properly means taking in nothing but water or other noncaloric fluids. Eating nothing but fruit for a day is really a restricted diet rather than a fast, but it is an easy introduction to the technique of limiting what you eat as a way of influencing your whole being, body, mind, and spirit.

In many cultures, dietary restriction is an aspect of religious observance: think of the Lenten prohibitions of Roman Catholics, the Yom Kippur fast of Jews, and the whole month of daytime abstinence from food that Muslims practice during Ramadan. Fasting also exists as an Eastern tradition. The Buddha tried it before he settled on meditation as the path to enlightenment, and Indian ascetics commonly use it today to help develop God-consciousness.

Fasting also has its enthusiasts among people interested in improving their health, people who may be not at all religious. It can be an effective technique, owing to a basic fact of physiology. The digestive organs are the largest and bulkiest in the body, and their routine operations consume large amounts of energy. The simple act of not eating, or eating only simple foods, frees up much of that energy for the body to use in healing. Animals naturally tend to stop eating at the onset of sickness, and humans who do the same often report that the course of sickness is shorter than expected as a result.

As a purely psychological discipline without religious connotation, dietary restriction can provide insight into the workings of the mind. Many people eat to satisfy emotional needs as much as to nourish their bodies. People commonly eat to allay anxiety, to try to fill inner emptiness resulting from lack of love and connection to others, and to anesthetize themselves against emotional pain. Some use involvement with food and eating as a way of filling time and distracting themselves. It is interesting to observe what happens when you seal yourself off from that escape route, when you deny the mind a familiar source of comfort. At the least, it can make you more appreciative of food and encourage you to eat more mindfully.

In this second half of the Eight-Week Program, I will give you some options for experimenting with dietary restriction and fasting. Even if you try them for the modest purpose of giving your digestive system a rest, I think you will find the experiences useful. This week you can, if you want, start with a fruit fast. Eat nothing but fresh fruit one day of the week, and drink as much water and herbal tea as you want. Fruit is not taxing to the digestive system, since it mostly provides natural sugars that are easily broken down and assimilated. It also gives you vitamins, minerals, and fiber—all good things. When you get into bed that evening, note how you feel. Do you feel hungry? deprived? virtuous? lighter? Note any effects on your energy and sense of well-being. If this experiment agrees with you, you might want to do a day of fruit fasting on a regular basis, or as an antidote to a period of eating heavily and unwisely.

A HEALING STORY:
THE POWER OF GINGER

I HAVE KNOWN Caron Smith since I was in medical school. She married one of my roommates, and we have all been friends ever since. Caron holds a Ph.D. in Chinese art and archeology, teaches those subjects at Bard Graduate Center for Studies in the Decorative Arts, has been on the staff of the Metropolitan Museum of Art, and now, at fifty-three, is curator and associate director of galleries at the Asia Society in New York. Perhaps it is in part her affinity for Chinese culture that makes her so receptive to ginger's therapeutic effects. This is what she tells me:

Eight years ago, in 1988, I think, I began to feel a certain stiffness in my hands, especially in the morning. I experienced no limitation of motion, just stiffness and achiness, which was really annoying. My mother's sisters all had osteoarthritis, so that was at the back of my mind. When I heard from you about the anti-inflammatory effect of ginger, I decided to give it a try. I began taking three capsules of powdered ginger (550 milligrams each) in the morning. After two to three months, I noticed a remission of the feeling in my hands.

I had also been having gastric distress at this time, which I think was due mostly to my irregular eating habits and maybe also to drinking a lot of coffee. As I began taking ginger regularly, this symptom also abated. And if I stopped the ginger, after three to four days I would notice a return of both the stiffness in my hands and the distress in my stomach. At one point I ran out of ginger, and because I was very busy, I did not buy any more for a month. There was a big difference, so I resolved to make it part of my daily regimen. I really began to look at it as a source of relief.

I eat ginger at every opportunity (especially pickled ginger with Japanese food). I recommend it to others. I remember reading that Confucius was never without ginger when he ate. It's the easiest remedy in the world to use, with no side effects. It's pungent; its flower is intoxicating. If I'd had a daughter, I think I would have named her Ginger.

10

Week Six

Projects

• Look over the information on tonics in the commentary. Decide on one that is appropriate for you and find out where to get it.
• Take a steam bath or sauna twice this week.

Diet

• Continue to eat fish twice this week and soy foods twice this week.
• Continue to eat broccoli at least twice.
• Add some cooked greens to your diet this week: collards, kale, chard, beet or mustard greens, for example. Recipe ideas begin on page 142.

Mental/Spiritual

• Extend your news fast to four days.
• Visit an art museum or try to view some work of art, sculpture, or architecture that you find beautiful and inspiring.
• Practice all the breathing exercises every day.

Optional

• Try a one-day "juice fast" this week: any amount of fruit and vegetable juices you care to drink, plus water and herbal tea. Take vitamin C but skip the other supplements on this day.

COMMENTARY

Projects

Your assignment this week is to inform yourself about tonics and begin thinking about using one.

The root meaning of the word "tonic" is "stretch." My definition of a tonic in the medical sense is a nontoxic, natural substance that has the ability to stretch or tone the body when used regularly over time. Athletes and fitness buffs are very familiar with muscle tone, but most people do not extend the concept of toning to internal organs and body functions. A particular problem that our culture has with the concept is that the whole idea of health tonics is disreputable, the result of associations with patent-medicine salesmen of the past and the opprobrium of the medical and scientific establishments toward this class of remedies. Yet, in ethnomedical traditions around the world, people hold tonic plants in the highest esteem, often paying more for them than for any sort of medicine.

Conventional medical doctors are suspicious of all treatments with general effects. Doctors and pharmaceutical companies have come to like drugs with highly specific actions—magic bullets. If a drug begins to work on too many different conditions, our scientists lose interest in it, because they think generality of action indicates absence of a specific pharmacological mechanism, throwing any observed benefit into the dubious realm of placebo responses and nonscience. I find this attitude to be limiting and unhelpful. I like to point out that in traditional Chinese medicine, which groups medicines into three categories called *superior, middle,* and *inferior,* it is the inferior ones that have specific effects on specific conditions. To the Chinese medical mind, the highest ideal of a remedy is one that works for everything—a panacea. It is in this superior category that the great tonics of Chinese medicine are found: ginseng, for example, and the woody mushroom known as *ling chih* (usually found here under its Japanese name, *reishi*).

Let me tell you a bit of the rich history of ginseng as an illustration of the effects of limiting conceptions in medical research and practice. Ginseng is obtained from the root of several species of slow-growing woodland plants. Two species provide most of the ginseng in commerce: *Panax ginseng,* native to East Asia and known as Asian ginseng, and *Panax quinquefolius,* native to eastern North America, known as American ginseng. By the way, the genus *Panax* takes its name from Panacea, a minor Greek goddess of healing, whose name translates as All-Heal; the plant was given that name by Chinese doctors who believed that its root is good for everything.

By the time Westerners first reached the Imperial Court in Peking in the sixteenth century, Asian ginseng was already priced extravagantly, since demand for this universal remedy exceeded supply, and the Chinese were always looking for new sources. Spanish Jesuits were the first Westerners to come, and the imperial bureaucrats recognized their utility at once. Here was a worldwide network of highly educated men who maintained communication with each other. The Chinese gave them samples of ginseng with the request that they be sent to all of their outposts in an effort to find new sources. Sometime in the seventeenth century, some of these samples reached a Jesuit mission in Quebec, where a similar plant did indeed grow in the woods. This was American ginseng, a plant not extensively used by Native Americans that was abundant throughout eastern North America. Eventually, samples of it were brought back to Peking, and eventually word came from the Forbidden City to "send as much as you can."

So began the commercialization of American ginseng for sale to an ever-demanding Chinese market. Harvesting of the roots reached such a level that within a century ginseng was extinct in eastern Canada, and the trade spread south to New England and New York, then westward with the settlers of the new land. Many pioneers made their living picking ginseng, or "seng," as they called it; Daniel Boone supported himself in this way, for example. Soon wild-ginseng stands in New England and New York suffered the same fate as those in Canada, and the more westerly populations were then threatened by overharvesting.

Now many Chinese people prefer American ginseng to their own species. A conventional Western doctor would probably say this was just a case of placebos' being greener on the other side of the ocean, but the two species actually have different properties: *P. ginseng* is more of a stimulant, and *P. quinquefolius* more of an "adaptogen," a term coined by a Russian scientist to designate ability to confer resistance to stress of all sorts. We Americans let our own native stands of this valuable and beneficial plant be harvested almost to extinction without taking any scientific interest in it, until consumers here began to learn about ginseng and buy it. Throughout the eighteenth and nineteenth centuries and for most of the twentieth, American pharmacologists and doctors ignored ginseng, and those Americans who knew the plant knew it only as something strange people far away paid money for. The obstacle to taking the plant seriously here as a natural medicine was that claims for general heal-all properties made our scientists think it was worthless, as far from a magic bullet as a remedy could be.

We now know that ginseng is full of biologically active compounds (ginsenosides) that work on the pituitary-adrenal axis. This hormonal influence could certainly account for many of the effects attributed to the root: its positive effect on the metabolism of skin, muscle, and bone, for example; its tendency to give people more energy, more sexual vigor, and more resistance. In Chinese medical philosophy, tonics are thought to work on the defensive sphere of function of the human body; anything that increases natural resistance would, of course, produce general effects and look like a panacea. I think tonics work directly on the healing system, increasing not only defensive capability but also the body's ability to repair itself, replace damaged structure, and regenerate new structure. I hope our scientists are finally beginning to take this important category of natural medicines seriously.

I have already encouraged you to become more familiar with two well-known tonic herbs—ginger and garlic, which should now be appearing regularly on your table as you enter Week Six of the Eight-Week Program. Green tea, introduced in Week Two, is another that I hope you have tried. Now I'd like to review for you some other natural products for you to consider. Before you complete the program, I want you to select one or two to experiment with. To give a tonic a fair test, you should take it every day for at least two months. In some cases the effect will be imperceptible but you will know that you are reducing certain health risks; in other cases the effect will be obvious, such as feeling increased energy.

As a way of introducing these products, let me tell you a bit about one currently promoted by the medical profession but not acknowledged to be a tonic: aspirin. Aspirin is a semisynthetic derivative of white-willow bark, meaning that chemists, a century ago, created it by making a small chemical change in salicylic acid, a natural constituent of willow (*Salix*). Willow-bark tea was and is a folk remedy for fever and pain among Native Americans and Europeans. It is weak, however, and purified salicylic acid, the active component, is too irritating to the stomach. Acetylsalicylic acid—aspirin—is both more potent and less irritating. Its three classical actions—antipyretic (fever-reducing), analgesic (pain-relieving), and anti-inflammatory—have made it one of the most widely used remedies in the world.

I have heard pharmacologists say that if aspirin were a new drug, just invented, it would stand little chance of FDA approval, because its actions are so general, and its toxicity, in overdose, so great. But as you now know, generality of action is a big advantage as I see it, making aspirin a candidate for admission to the superior category of medicines, and few other drugs have such an excellent safety record, considering how many people have taken it and how often since its invention.

Researchers keep discovering new effects of aspirin that lead doctors to recommend it to everyone, not just people with fevers, headaches, and arthritis. It keeps platelets from clumping, reducing the risk of blood clots and therefore of heart attacks and strokes. It reduces risk of colon cancer. It reduces risk of esophageal cancer—one of the worst forms of malignancy, with a dismal prognosis despite treatment. It reduces the risk of lung cancer. And it may reduce the risk of Alzheimer's disease. How aspirin accomplishes these miracles, we do not fully know. It works on the prostaglandin system, which I described earlier in this book,* and through it may have profound influence on cell growth and differentiation throughout the body. Moreover, lower doses of aspirin may work better as a tonic and preventive than higher, which challenges the conventional wisdom that more of a good thing must be better. A standard aspirin tablet contains 5 grains—that is, 325 milligrams—of acetylsalicylic acid. Maximal tonic benefit may come from as little as 80 milligrams a day. (I currently take 162 milligrams—that is, two low-dose tablets or half a regular tablet—and I take it with food to spare my stomach unnecessary irritation. I recommend a low-dose aspirin regimen to many patients and friends, and I would like you to consider using it, too, especially if you are at risk for any of the diseases I listed above.

---

* See page 35.

I will also ask my colleagues to begin thinking of aspirin as a true tonic, even though it is neither completely natural nor completely non-toxic. This request makes obvious that I am quite willing to use pharmaceutical drugs in appropriate ways. Also, if doctors will begin to see one of their most familiar remedies in this new perspective, it might be easier for them to appreciate the tonic nature of more exotic ones.

Here are eight other tonics for you to consider:

ASHWAGANDHA

Ashwagandha is an herbal remedy from the Ayurvedic tradition of India, the root of a plant (*Withania somnifera*) in the nightshade family. The species name *somnifera* means "sleep-bearing," suggesting that the plant is sedative, but in Ayurvedic medicine it is valued as a general tonic and restorer of male sexual potency—attributions similar to those for Asian ginseng. Ashwagandha is little-known in the West at the moment, certainly much less well known than ginseng; it is also much less expensive.

Recent animal research shows the stress-protective effects of ashwagandha and ginseng to be comparable, and a few clinical reports that I have reviewed make me think that the therapeutic potential of this plant is great. (See page 146 for a dramatic example.) Of course, serious clinical trials need to be conducted, but in the meantime, ashwagandha is nontoxic, affordable, and available for use. You will find capsules and extracts in health-food stores, often in the Ayurvedic herbal sections that are beginning to appear in those stores, as that form of traditional medicine makes inroads here. Follow the dosage recommended on the label, and give it a good two-month trial.

ASTRAGALUS

Astragalus is a large genus in the pea family, some species of which are toxic to livestock. (Locoweed of the American Southwest is an astragalus.) But the toxins are only in the above-ground parts, and this tonic comes from the root of a nontoxic Chinese species, *A. membranaceus*. The plant is a perennial with long, fibrous roots, native to North China and Inner Mongolia, sold in both wild and cultivated forms. Chinese pharmacies sell bundles of thin root-slices that resemble tongue depressors and have a sweet taste. These are simmered in medicinal soups, the slices being removed before serving because they are too tough to chew. Chinese pharmacies also sell many preparations of astragalus, both singly and in combination with other herbs. These are popular remedies for the prevention and treatment of colds and flus. You will find similar products in herb stores here.

Practitioners of traditional Chinese medicine consider astragalus a true tonic that can strengthen debilitated patients and increase resistance to disease in general. In contemporary Chinese medicine, it is also a chief component of *fu zheng* therapy, a combination herbal treatment designed to restore immune function in cancer patients undergoing chemotherapy and radiation therapy. Research in China has demonstrated increased survival in patients receiving both herbal and Western therapies, as well as protection from the immunosuppressive effects of the latter. I commonly recommend astragalus to cancer patients; it will not interfere with the conventional therapies. Studies in the West confirm that astragalus enhances immune function by increasing activity of several kinds of white blood cells and boosting production of antibodies and interferon, the body's own antiviral agent.

If you feel you lack energy and vitality, have depressed immunity, and get too many colds, consider going on a course of astragalus. Follow dosage recommendations on labels.

CORDYCEPS

Known in China as the "caterpillar fungus," *Cordyceps sinensis* is a peculiar mushroom that parasitizes the bodies of certain moth larvae. Fine threads of the fungal organism penetrate the living body of a larva, killing it and mummifying it. The mushroom then sends up its fruiting body, a slender stalk with a swollen end that will release spores. Cordyceps is found in mountainous regions of China and Tibet and is now much cultivated, because it is in great demand as a powerful tonic and restorative, believed to increase physical stamina, mental energy, sexual vigor, and longevity. It has a particular reputation for improving athletic performance, perhaps by increasing cardiac output, and I have a number of reports from runners who say it has improved their times in races. In China, cordyceps is considered safe and gentle, useful for both men and women of any age and state of health, even the most infirm.

Chinese people buy whole dried cordyceps (including the mummified larvae and fungal fruit bodies) and simmer them in soups and stews made from duck and chicken to create medicinal foods. You can do the same (see appendix for a source), or buy powdered cordyceps for making tea, liquid extracts that may include other Chinese herbs, or encapsulated forms. For general weakness, take it once a day, following dosage advice on the product. For health maintenance, in the absence of specific problems, take it once or twice a week.

DONG QUAI

The root of *Angelica sinensis,* a plant in the carrot family, dong quai is a popular blood-building tonic and circulatory stimulant in traditional Chinese medicine, but in this century Westerners have discovered its usefulness as a general tonic for women. Many Western herbalists and naturopaths and some physicians now recommend it for disorders of the female reproductive system, especially for irregular or difficult menstruation. Chinese doctors recognize its ability to tone the uterus and balance female hormonal chemistry, but they think of dong quai as beneficial for both sexes and often include it in tonic formulas for men, combined with ginseng. In men it is supposed to help build muscle and blood.

Dong quai is nontoxic and effective. I have frequently recommended it to women experiencing menstrual problems or menopausal symptoms and to those who lack energy, all with good results. You can easily find it in health-food stores in tincture or capsule form. If you want to experiment with it, try taking two capsules of the root twice a day, or one dropperful of the tincture in a little water twice a day.

GINSENG

Since I have already written at length about ginseng, I need only give you some practical advice about it. Many forms of ginseng are on the market, from whole dried roots to ginseng brandies, candies, wines, teas, and a multitude of liquid and solid extracts. I must warn you that some of these products contain little or no ginseng. Whenever a medicinal plant is scarce, expensive, and in great demand, imitation and adulterated products will abound. *Panax* (both the Asian and American species) owes its beneficial effects to ginsenosides, unusual compounds not found elsewhere in nature. If ginseng products are real, they must contain ginsenosides, the more the better, so, unless you are buying whole roots (which are unmistakable once you have seen them), stick to standardized products whose labels state the ginsenoside content.

Ginseng is generally safe, but the Asian variety *can raise blood pressure in some individuals, as well as cause irritability and insomnia.* If you experience these effects, lower the dose or switch to American ginseng, which may be better as a first choice unless you want to feel stimulated or are a man looking for increased sexual drive. Both Asian and American ginseng may have estrogenic activity that would argue against their use by women with hormonal imbalances or with estrogen-dependent ailments (uterine fibroids, fibrocystic breasts, endometriosis, and breast, uterine, and cervical cancer).

Whole roots are meant to be chopped and simmered at length into a medicinal tea. It is easier to take liquid extracts, capsules, or tablets. One brand of standardized Asian-ginseng extract, made by a Swiss method, is now available in drugstores throughout the world. Labels of these products will indicate proper dosages. I recommend ginseng frequently to people with low vitality or weakness due to chronic illness or old age. Most people who try it report that they are happy with its effects and plan to continue to take it.

MAITAKE

Maitake is the Japanese name for a mushroom, *Grifola frondosa,* that is both edible and medicinal. American mushroom-hunters know it as "hen of the woods," because it grows in big clusters, weighing up to one hundred pounds, at the bases of trees or stumps, clusters that resemble the fluffed tailfeathers of a nesting hen. In the early 1980s, Japanese scientists began to cultivate maitake on sawdust. The cultivated form is now sold in supermarkets throughout Japan; it looks like a dark-gray floral bouquet, except instead of flowers it is made up of many overlapping fan-shaped mushroom caps. Mushroom growers here are just beginning to produce maitake, a very tasty mushroom with remarkable tonic effects, especially on the immune system.

Research in Japan indicates that maitake has significant anticancer, antiviral, and immune-enhancing properties. It may also reduce blood pressure and blood sugar. I recommend it often to people with cancer, AIDS, and other immune-deficiency states, chronic fatigue syndrome, chronic hepatitis, and environmental illnesses that may represent toxic overloads. You can buy the dried mushroom (which should be reconstituted in water, then cooked with rice or in stir-fries), tablets of it, or liquid extract. My tonic of choice at the moment is a liquid extract called Maitake D-fraction, which concentrates the immune-boosting constituents (see appendix for a source). I take five drops in water three times a day, and since I've been doing so I almost never get colds, even though my children and their friends are constantly bringing colds into our house. If you are lucky enough to get the actual mushrooms, fresh or dried, eat them frequently; otherwise follow the recommended dosage on the products you buy.

MILK THISTLE

This remarkable remedy comes from the tradition of European folk medicine. It is the seed of a robust, spiny plant, *Silybum marianum,* that has great liver-protective properties. An extract of the seed, silymarin, enhances metabolism of liver cells and protects them from toxic injury. Conventional medicine has nothing comparable to offer patients with liver problems. And milk-thistle products are completely nontoxic and cheap.

I recommend this tonic for all heavy users of alcohol and pharmaceutical drugs that are hard on the liver, including cancer patients undergoing chemotherapy. (It will not interfere with chemotherapy.) I also recommend it to patients with chronic hepatitis and abnormal liver function from any cause. When added to a sensible regimen of dietary and lifestyle change, it can return liver function to normal after several months of regular use. If you work with toxic chemicals or feel you have suffered toxic exposures from any source, take milk thistle for a while. It will help your body recover from any harm.

You will find this remedy in all health-food stores. My preference—always with herbal products—is to rely on standardized extracts. Follow the suggested dosage on the label of the product you buy, or take two tablets or capsules twice a day. You can stay on milk thistle indefinitely.

REISHI

Reishi is a mushroom, *Ganoderma lucidum,* that grows on trees, has a surface that appears lacquered, and is one of the most important tonics in the traditional medicine of China and Japan, particularly esteemed for extending longevity. Reishi is a purely medicinal mushroom, not a culinary one, both because it is hard and woody and because it tastes very bitter. But it is nontoxic and has been the subject of a surprising amount of scientific research, both in Asia and the West. Although most of the research has been in animals, the results are so promising that I think human studies will soon follow. Like maitake and other related mushroom species, reishi improves immune function and inhibits the growth of some malignant tumors. Additionally, it shows significant anti-inflammatory effect, reduces allergic responsiveness, and protects the liver.

Because it is easily cultivated, reishi is widely available and not too expensive. If you don't mind the bitterness, you can make tea of the ground mushroom; in some products it is mixed with other tonic mushrooms that improve the taste. Or you can buy reishi tablets. Follow the recommended dosage, and take reishi every day for at least two months to see what it can do for you.

SIBERIAN GINSENG

The last tonic I will tell you about comes from the root of a large, spiny shrub, *Eleutherococcus senticosus,* native to North China and Siberia. It is one of the most widely used herbs in the world, so much in demand that authentic material may be hard to find. Also known as "spiny" and "eleuthero" ginseng, this species is a relative of true (*Panax*) ginseng. Soviet scientists discovered its adaptogenic properties in the course of searching for ginseng substitutes, and as news of its benefits spread, many Soviet athletes and military personnel began to use it to increase physical performance and endurance.

The stress-protective effects of Siberian ginseng are well documented in both animal and human studies, as is its ability to enhance immune function. The active components are a distinctive group of compounds called *eleutherosides,* and unless Siberian-ginseng products specify their eleutheroside content, you are probably not getting the real thing. I find it to be a reliable tonic with general restorative effects, especially useful for people who lack energy and vitality. It is nontoxic and can be used safely over long periods of time. Take two capsules or tablets of a standardized extract twice a day, unless the label on the product you buy specifies otherwise.

. . .

With this information you can plan a trial of a tonic that you can start in the last week of the Eight-Week Program. Pick one or two that interest you and seem suited to your needs, then inquire about their availability and decide how you will use them. Tonics are allies in your progress toward optimum health. Learn how to take advantage of these gifts from nature.

Diet

I would like you to add some cooked greens to your diet this week. If you have not discovered the delights of these healthy vegetables, you may find this assignment challenging. I would not have considered eating greens when I was growing up, and tasting some of the ghastly versions served to me in school and hospital cafeterias confirmed my childhood aversion. You may have had the same experience, which is too bad, because dark, leafy greens are full of natural agents that can protect health, and they are too often missing from our diets.

Greens are high in vitamins and minerals, including iron and calcium in forms that the body can absorb and use more readily than supplements. For example, they are a major source of folic acid (folate), a B vitamin that regulates protein metabolism and offers significant protection against coronary heart disease. ("Folate" and "foliage" share the same root.) In other cultures, cooked greens appear with great regularity at most meals, even with breakfast in traditional Japanese cuisine. In general, Asians are very good about eating their greens, and have many varieties to choose from. One teaching of yoga dietetics is that optimum health requires eating freshly cooked greens at least once a day. In the American South, people eat greens more often than in other parts of the country, but they generally drown them in fat, often bacon grease. If you have only met greens that were cooked to death, you are in for a pleasant surprise when you try the recipes below.

Some greens have strong tastes that some people dislike; beet greens and chard, for example, both contain oxalic acid, which accounts for a sharp flavor. Often older leaves have more of this flavor than younger ones, and some varieties are stronger-tasting than others. I grow a white beet in my garden whose leaves taste mild at all stages of maturity, and I only eat young chard. On the other hand, I find kale to be generally mild and good-tasting, as long as it is prepared properly.

Improper preparation can result in unappetizing textures as well as colors and flavors. If you do not remove the tough central stalks of big leaves, you will wind up with pieces of them on your plate and in your mouth. Cutting leaves into shreds or bite-size pieces makes them more appealing. I am not fond of thick, curly varieties of kale, but I love smooth, tender ones. If you do not like your greens straight, you can try mixing them with pasta, potatoes, rice, or beans. They are easy to prepare, and I encourage you to try them. I believe that including these foods in your diet will reduce risks of cancer and heart disease, improve digestion, and help protect your healing system from toxic injury.

Here is a recipe for a light soup containing three tonic herbs—garlic, ginger, and astragalus. It also has onion and shiitake to lower cholesterol, and vegetables rich in antioxidants.

☙ *Tonic Soup* ❧

8 cups vegetable stock (see pages 89–91)
1 tablespoon olive oil
1 onion, diced
4–8 cloves garlic, minced
1 1-inch piece of fresh gingerroot, peeled and finely chopped
1 cup sliced carrots
1 slice astragalus root
1 cup shiitake mushrooms (fresh or reconstituted), sliced
1 cup broccoli flowerets

1. Bring the vegetable broth to a boil in a large pot.
2. Meanwhile, heat the olive oil in a skillet and add the onion, garlic, and ginger. Sauté over low heat until soft and aromatic.
3. Add contents of skillet to broth along with carrots, astragalus root, and shiitake mushrooms.
4. Simmer, covered, 1 hour.
5. Add the broccoli flowerets in the last 5 minutes, and remove astragalus before serving.

And here are some of my favorite recipes using greens:

✌ *Kale with Potatoes* ✊

1 pound medium red potatoes
4 cups shredded kale (see procedure below)
2 tablespoons olive oil
1 large onion, chopped
salt to taste

1. The potatoes can be prepared in advance and refrigerated. Boil them until tender. Peel while hot, then cool in cold water and drain. Cut into thick slices.

2. Wash the kale, drain, and remove the stems and midribs. Stack leaves, roll up lengthwise, and shred crosswise. (Always choose kale that is not wilted, with good color. I much prefer smooth varieties to curly ones; my favorite is red Russian.)

3. In a large skillet, heat the olive oil and add the onion. Sauté over medium-high heat, stirring, until onion just begins to brown.

4. Add kale, tossing it about until it all wilts. Reduce heat to medium and stir-fry kale for 5 minutes more.

5. Add the potatoes and cook until they are heated through. Season to taste with salt and serve.

✌ *Pasta with Greens* ✊

1/2 cup sundried tomatoes
1 pound dried pasta (penne, rigatoni, twists, etc.)
1 pound greens (collards, kale, beet greens, chard, or a mixture of these)
2 tablespoons olive oil
1 large onion, thinly sliced
1/2 teaspoon hot red-pepper flakes
2–4 cloves garlic, minced
1 tablespoon dried basil
2 tablespoons capers
grated Parmesan cheese (optional)

1. Soak the sundried tomatoes in hot water till soft, about 10 minutes. Drain, cut into pieces, and reserve.

2. Begin cooking the pasta.

3. While pasta is cooking, prepare greens: wash, drain, remove all coarse stems and midribs, then chop coarsely and reserve.

4. Heat the olive oil in a skillet, add the onion and red-pepper flakes, and sauté over medium high heat.

5. When onions begin to color, add the tomatoes and chopped greens, tossing well to wilt. Mash in the garlic, add basil, and cook for 5 minutes. Add capers with a little of their liquid.

6. Drain the pasta and mix with vegetables. Serve with grated Parmesan cheese if desired.

↝ *Beet Greens and Tofu* ↜

1 cup tofu cubes (see procedure below)
1 pound beet greens
1 tablespoon canola oil
1 medium onion, chopped
1 clove garlic, mashed
reduced-sodium soy sauce or teriyaki sauce to taste

1. If you use fresh tofu for this easy and surprisingly good dish, drain it, slice it 1/2-inch thick, place the slices on a dish towel or layers of paper towel, cover with another cloth or paper towel, then place a board on top and weight the board with a few heavy cans or a pot of water. Press the tofu slices for 1 hour, then remove and cut into 1/2-inch cubes. You can also use baked, pressed tofu, in which case you just need to cut it into cubes. Either way, you will want to end up with 1 cup of tofu cubes.

2. Wash the beet greens, drain, remove stems, and shred.

3. Heat the canola oil in a skillet and add the onion. Sauté over medium-high heat until onion is translucent, then add the tofu and continue cooking until tofu begins to color.

4. Add the beet greens and garlic. Stir-fry until greens are cooked, about 5 minutes.

5. Season with the soy sauce or teriyaki sauce and cook for another minute to blend flavors. Serve over brown rice.

ᴥ *Curried Greens* ᴥ

1 pound spinach, kale, collards, or beet greens
2 cloves garlic, minced
2–3 tablespoons curry powder
1 cup finely chopped tomatoes (fresh or canned)
1 tablespoon tomato paste
1 tablespoon dark-brown sugar
1 tablespoon canola oil
1 cup onion, finely diced
3/4 pound potatoes, peeled and cubed
1/4 cup chopped fresh cilantro (optional)

1. Wash and drain greens, removing any coarse stems and midribs. Cut into 1/2-inch strips.

2. In a bowl, mix together the garlic, curry powder, tomatoes, tomato paste, and sugar.

3. Heat the canola oil in a skillet and sauté onion over medium-high heat until it begins to brown. Add the spice-and-tomato mixture, mix well, and cook for a few minutes.

4. Add the potatoes and 2 cups water.

5. Mix well, bring to a boil, reduce heat, cover, and cook for 10 minutes.

6. Add greens and cook for 10 minutes more, or until potatoes are done. Correct seasoning. Garnish with the chopped fresh cilantro if desired.

ᴥ *Hot and Sour Greens* ᴥ

1 pound greens (bok choy, kale, collards, or Chinese cabbage)
2 teaspoons canola oil
2 large cloves garlic, minced
1/4 teaspoon hot red-pepper flakes
1/4 teaspoon dry mustard powder
2 tablespoons rice vinegar
1 teaspoon soy sauce
1 teaspoon light-brown sugar

1. Wash and drain greens, remove any tough stems, and slice leaves into 1/2-inch shreds. (If using bok choy or Chinese cabbage, trim off the end, slice stems 1/4 inch thick and leaves 1/2 inch thick.)

2. Heat the canola oil in a skillet over medium heat. Add the garlic and red-pepper flakes and stir-fry for 1 minute.

3. Add the greens along with the mustard and stir to coat with the spices.

4. Combine the rice vinegar, soy sauce, and sugar and add to skillet. Cook covered over medium heat until vegetables are tender, about 5 minutes.

Mental/Spiritual

You have a fun assignment this week: appreciate a work of art. Just as music and the natural beauty of flowers and parks can raise your spirits, so can beautiful paintings, sculpture, and architecture. Pay a visit this week to a favorite work of art, whether a painting in a museum, a favorite building, or a statue. Just admire it, letting it please your senses and nourish your nonphysical being.

Optional

Restrict yourself during one day to juices, both fruit and vegetable. If you can prepare the juices yourself or buy them freshly prepared, they will taste better and give you more nutrients, because juice deteriorates quickly on exposure to air. Drink as much juice as you want, along with plenty of water and herbal tea if you desire. Limiting your diet to fruit and vegetable juice is a way to give your digestive system a good rest.

A Healing Story:
A Testimonial to Ashwagandha
(and Ayurveda)

I MET Dr. Patricia Ammon, a family-practice doctor from Ouray, Colorado, at a conference on botanical medicine in March 1996. When she told me she had had multiple sclerosis I was surprised, because she looked completely well. I asked her to write down her story.

Having graduated from a family-practice residency in 1991 at the age of thirty-four, I was thrilled to be embarking on my new career as a physician in the Telluride (Colorado) Medical Clinic. My husband and I moved a house trailer to our dream land on Horsefly Mesa with a spectacular view of the San Juan Mountains, settled down to work hard, build our dream house, and live happily ever after. During the winter of 1991–92, I noticed more fatigue than I had ever felt as a resident. Our house is well off the highway, and the county does not maintain the county road, which we didn't consider a problem, as we are both avid cross-country skiers. By April 1992, after five months of skiing the mile to our home, it became apparent that I was having difficulty with the uphill part of the trail. I blamed this on the increasing stress I perceived in my job.

I decided I needed more time off and left the Telluride clinic to work at an emergency clinic in another town, where I had eight twenty-four-hour shifts a month. Through the summer I continued to experience fatigue and developed a fairly profound depression. My family physician recommended counseling and antidepressants. By fall 1992, I was having numbness in my left leg and was more depressed than ever, despite high doses of antidepressants.

In January 1993, I finally saw a neurologist at my family physician's insistence; I was too depressed and drugged to think clearly. An MRI scan showed multiple sclerosis beyond a doubt. I got up from the MRI table, talked to the radiologist, who was a friend, and went and purchased a one-way ticket to Hawaii to visit a friend I trained with in residency. She is a practicing Buddhist who was able to teach me some yoga and meditation techniques. I returned home after three weeks and, unwisely, went right back to work in the emergency department. By June 1993, I was having numbness in my left foot and hand, and right side of my face. My handwriting, which had always been good, became unreadable.

In July of that year, I went to an MS center for evaluation and was advised to have four days of inpatient treatment with high-dose steroids. I was scared but felt so miserable that I agreed to the plan. I spent four days in a hospital in Denver receiving 1 gram of intravenous Solu-Medrol a day, which made me quite psychotic. After I came home I was much worse than before. I gained weight, couldn't sleep, and had to decrease my work hours, often not being able to finish my shift. The depression was almost unbearable. I could walk around the emergency department and my home but could not walk more than one-eighth of a mile continuously. Prior to the steroids I felt bad, but at least I could walk up to a mile a day, and I slept OK.

In the fall of 1993, I visited Paul Curlee, M.D., an internal-medicine physician on the faculty where I did my residency. I knew he practiced Ayurvedic medicine [the traditional medicine of India] but had paid little attention to this as a resident—there was so much else to learn. Paul suggested some yoga exercises and a combination herbal treatment. In October 1993, I consulted another Ayurvedic practitioner, Nancy Lonsdorf, M.D., who had just completed a book on the subject. Nancy took my pulse, did an exam, and told me I had a deep imbalance of vata [one of three humors recognized in Ayurveda]. She suggested pancha karma [a detoxification regimen, consisting of restricted diet, oil massages, steam baths, and herbal treatments].

That November, I went to the Ayurvedic clinic in Fairfield, Iowa, for pancha karma and also learned transcendental meditation. After one week I was walking at least two miles a day, sleeping much better, and feeling better than I had in ten years. My husband

and friends told me I looked two to three years younger than before I went. I was started on some Ayurvedic herbs, the main one being ashwagandha. I changed my diet to mostly vegetarian with some fish, and practiced yoga regularly.

From November 1993 through February 1995, I went back to the Fairfield clinic four more times, each time feeling better and better. I took a physicians' training course in Ayurveda, as much for my own health as anything. I was able to open a family-practice clinic in Ouray and start up an integrative practice.

In November 1995, I found a chiropractor in Boulder, John Douillard, who had opened an Ayurvedic clinic closer to home. He practices a traditional form of Ayurveda, which I find superior to the form I learned. Under his supervision, I continue to take ashwagandha every day and continue to feel quite well. I walk at least two miles a day, cross-country ski up to ten miles at a time with minimal fatigue, and I have no hint of depression. I no longer practice transcendental meditation; instead I use a combination of mindfulness meditation, breathing exercises, and contemplative prayer. I also recently learned some Qi Gong [Chinese energy-healing] practices that I find very enjoyable.

I now regard the diagnosis of MS as a blessing in disguise. It brought me to a much more spiritual path and reminded me that my task is to be a healer, not just a physician, and, most importantly, a healer to myself. I have endeavored to learn about botanical medicine, Ayurveda, Chinese medicine, and the role of spirituality in everything, an orientation I may not have come to without the diagnosis. It is very exciting to be part of the shifting attitude toward health care in this country, both personally and professionally.

11

Week Seven

Projects

• Do some kind of service work this week, such as volunteering for a few hours at a hospital or charitable organization or helping someone you know who is disabled or shut in—any activity in which you give some of your time and energy to help others.
• Continue the steam baths or saunas, twice this week if possible.

Diet

• Continue eating as before: at least two meals of fish and two of soy protein, generous servings of fruits, vegetables, whole grains, ginger, and garlic, and cooked greens twice this week.

Exercise

• Increase the aerobic walk to forty minutes, five days of the week.

Mental/Spiritual

• Reach out to resume connection with someone from whom you are estranged.
• Make time for flowers, music, and art.
• Increase the Relaxing Breath to eight cycles, twice a day.

Optional

• For a fast day this week, drink only fruit juice, water, and herbal tea. Take vitamin C but skip the other supplements on this day.

COMMENTARY

Projects

Your new project this week sounds simple, but it touches on a profound subject that is very relevant to health: your sense of self in relation to others.

As a way of introducing this topic, let me recount the story of a patient who once consulted me. Richard H. was forty-six years old when he came to my office. His manner was superficially engaging and pleasant, but I quickly sensed an underlying sadness and desperation about him. He had two chief complaints: chronic back pain and lack of energy. Both problems were of long duration, and I was at the end of a long list of practitioners he had visited over the years, none of whom had given him any solutions. Richard's back had bothered him on and off ever since he had injured it playing tennis almost ten years before. Orthopedists told him his X-rays and scans showed no significant structural problems, and the drugs and injections they prescribed had not helped. Nor had acupuncture, chiropractic, soaks in therapy pools, or yoga, although he had put a lot of time and money into all of them. Richard described the pain as "nagging," "constant," and "something I live with every day." He was convinced it had a physical basis that had eluded the doctors and therapists he had seen.

His other symptom—lack of energy—had crept up on him without a clear beginning, but now it interfered with his daily living, making it hard for him to focus on his work as an accountant, to exercise, or to do much with his evenings, which he usually spent by himself at home, watching television, reading, or "just crashing early, because I can't do anything else." Richard had divorced five years before and had not found another long-term relationship. He had no children. When I asked him about friends in his life, he replied, "Yes, I have friends," but when I questioned him more closely, I found out that these were mostly college friends, now living elsewhere and not frequently seen.

Richard's medical history revealed a number of other symptoms—headaches, hay fever, unexplained episodes of itching, and occasional stomach upsets—though none of these seemed serious to me or indicative of any underlying physical disease. His body was in reasonably good shape, yet something was clearly wrong. He was not living in a state of balance, and although many doctors would have said his health was fine, I thought he was on a downward slide that could eventually result in disease.

In my notes, I wrote, "Impression—Disconnection Syndrome," a diagnosis of my own invention, not recognized by most of my colleagues, one that lacks a numerical code that would make it official in the ICD (the International Classification of Diseases), the compendium of recognized disease conditions used by insurers and managed-care facilities. I am convinced of its reality, however, and identify it with increasing frequency in patients in our culture. And I do see it as a precursor of illness on the physical level, one that can over time derange the functioning of the cardiovascular system, the immune system, the endocrine system, and physiology in general.

In one way, Richard was lucky: despite his having seen a number of practitioners, he had avoided the trap of becoming a professional patient, whose life revolves around visits to doctors and trials of therapies. With his complaints and history, he was made to order for one of the fashionable diagnoses of today—chronic fatigue syndrome or fibromyalgia, for example—and for being taken advantage of by both conventional and alternative doctors. The orthopedist might have pushed him toward surgery, or Richard might have become a regular visitor to a chronic-pain clinic or been sent to endless physical therapy or put on long and costly rounds of electroacupuncture, intravenous vitamin infusions, magnet therapy, or countless other alternative treatments with little rationale to support them. All of this effort would have been directed to his physical body, but that was not where the cause of his discomfort lay, at least not yet.

Richard had gone to a marriage counselor during the year preceding his divorce and had done a few sessions of psychotherapy in the months following that event, but he was not very aware of his own feelings and not comfortable with discussing them. Although he was willing to consider the psychological dimension of his symptoms, like many people today he thought that back pain meant a problem in his back and fatigue meant something wrong with his immune system.

I assured him that his immune system was probably fine and explained to him that back pain—one of the commonest complaints that bring patients to doctors—has a very poor correlation with structural abnormalities. It is possible to find patients whose X-rays and CT and MRI scans look so bad that radiologists cannot imagine that these people could stand on their feet, yet the patients are free of pain. It is possible to find other patients who are totally disabled by back pain and have perfectly normal-looking spines on X-rays and scans. What does this say about the nature of back pain? At the very least it suggests that an abnormal physical finding should not, by itself, be used as justification for removal of a disk, laminectomy, or other drastic, invasive, and expensive procedure.

"Then what do you think is wrong with me?" he asked.

"I think you are disconnected," I replied. "You have no meaningful connections in your life, not to a mate, a lover, friends, your work, a hobby, a pet, or, really, anything beyond yourself and your symptoms. That is not healthy."

Human beings are highly social, communal animals. We are meant to live in families, tribes, and communities, and when we lack those connections we suffer. Yet many people pride themselves on their independence and habitually distance themselves from others. Some may indulge in isolation as a defensive strategy, possibly developed in reaction to painful emotional experiences in childhood. Others may never have learned how to connect meaningfully to anyone or anything beyond themselves. Of course, most people need experiences of solitude as well, some more than others, but if solitude is not balanced by connectedness, it is often productive of illness, first on the spiritual level, then the mental/emotional level, and finally crystallizing into the physical structure of the body. Those familiar with the philosophy of traditional Chinese medicine will recognize an analogy here. Chinese doctors say that all visible illness—illness of the body, of physical form—is preceded by invisible illness, that is, by illness of spirit, of the circulation of energy through the body. This is why I told Richard that he was not yet sick in the Western-medical sense but was likely to become so if he did not correct what was missing in his life.

People who are married, have children, and seem quite involved with the world can nonetheless suffer from Disconnection Syndrome and its long-range detrimental effect on health. Disconnection is an inner experience; the suffering it brings can be all the more intense when it occurs in the midst of a life apparently full of other people. The essential, inner, experiential problem is self-absorption, failure to recognize other beings as meaningful and worthy of attention. I do not know for sure that our culture is worse in this regard than others, but my experiences in Japan and traditional societies in the Third World make me suspect that it is. Western, industrialized society has substituted the nuclear family for the extended family, glorifies individualism and independence, and fosters a spirit of Every Man for Himself in many of its endeavors. This creates a deep, unsatisfied longing in people that may be at the root of much of our social malaise—the prevalence of addiction to drugs that numb feelings, for example, the growth of gangs among our youth, and rising violence everywhere.

I do know for sure that connectedness is necessary to well-being. You can eat as much salmon and broccoli as you can, take antioxidants for the rest of your life, breathe terrifically, and walk all over the earth, but if you are disconnected, you will not achieve optimum health.

I gave Richard a number of suggestions for changing his life, including working with a therapist to get at the root cause of his isolation, getting a puppy to love and care for (he had not had a pet since he was a child), finding a hobby that would involve him with a group, and doing some service work.

Service means helping others, giving of your time and energy to improve the welfare of others, without expectation of any return, whether of spiritual merit, admiration, or a sense of being virtuous. It is a practical demonstration of one's awareness that we are all connected as well as a tool for developing that awareness.

When the Dalai Lama accepted the Nobel Peace Prize in 1989, he said:

> The realization that we are all basically the same human beings, who seek happiness and try to avoid suffering, is very helpful in developing a sense of brotherhood and sisterhood—a warm feeling of love and compassion for others. This, in turn, is essential if we are to survive in this ever-shrinking world we live in. For if we each selfishly pursue only what we believe to be our own interest, without caring about the needs of others, we not only may end up harming others, but also ourselves. This fact has become very clear

during the course of this century. We know that to wage a nuclear war today, for example, would be a form of suicide; or that to pollute the air or the oceans, in order to achieve some short-term benefit, would be to destroy the very basis for our survival. As individuals and nations are becoming increasingly interdependent we have no other choice than to develop what I call a sense of universal responsibility. . . .

Responsibility does not only lie with the leaders of our countries or with those who have been appointed or elected to do a particular job. It lies with each of us individually. Peace, for example, starts within each one of us. When we have inner peace, we can be at peace with those around us. When our community is in a state of peace, it can share that peace with neighboring communities, and so on. When we feel love and kindness towards others, it not only makes others feel loved and cared for, but it helps us also to develop inner happiness and peace. And there are ways in which we can consciously work to develop feelings of love and kindness. For some of us, the most effective way to do so is through religious practice. For others it may be nonreligious practice. What is important is that we each make a sincere effort to take seriously our responsibility for each other. . . .

Service work is a common religious practice—think of the various charitable orders in the Roman Catholic Church, for example—but as a nonreligious practice it can equally qualify as a "sincere effort to take seriously our responsibility for each other."

Human suffering is boundless. There is no way that any individual, through however many good deeds, will lessen it significantly in its totality. But by devoting some of your time and energy to helping other individuals, you can make a difference in how you feel as well as how they feel, and that difference may translate into increased inner happiness and peace, and therefore into improved health. As a happier, healthier, and more peaceful individual, you will naturally stimulate those qualities in people around you.

Even if you consider yourself very well connected, have a loving family, never kick your dog, and frequently write checks to charities, you can benefit from the project I am asking you to undertake this week. I want you to think of some way you can be of service to at least one other person. You could give several hours of volunteer work to a community organization, for example, or help a disadvantaged person in some way, or teach someone a skill that you have, or entertain someone who is sick or shut in. The possibilities are myriad, and I will leave it to you to explore them. Remember: service work is a way of developing and demonstrating your sense of universal connectedness with other human beings. It is, truly, its own reward, and I have included it in the Eight-Week Program because I consider it one more piece of the whole picture of health.

Diet

Here are a few more recipes for you to try:

∽ *Lentil Soup* ∽

1 pound green lentils
1 Turkish bay leaf (or 1/3 California bay leaf)
3 large carrots, peeled and sliced
2 stalks celery, sliced
1 large onion, thinly sliced
1 tablespoon olive oil
2 cups crushed tomatoes or tomato puree
salt and vinegar (red-wine or balsamic) to taste
8 tofu wieners (optional)

1. Pick over the lentils to remove any stones, dirt, and other foreign objects. Wash them well in cold water. Place in large pot with enough cold water to cover lentils by 6 inches and add the bay leaf. Bring to a boil, skim off foam, lower heat, and boil gently, partially covered, until lentils are just tooth-tender, about 45–60 minutes.

2. Add the carrots, celery, and onion. Cook partially covered until carrots are tender, about 20–30 minutes.

3. Add the olive oil and tomatoes. Simmer, partially covered, until lentils become very creamy and soft, at least 1 hour more.

Stir occasionally and add boiling water if necessary to prevent sticking.

4. Flavor with salt and vinegar to taste, and remove bay leaf before serving. Optional: add sliced tofu wieners during the last hour of cooking.

✄ *Vegetarian Chili* ✄

1 pound Anasazi beans (or pintos)
2 large onions, sliced
2 tablespoons olive oil
1 tablespoon mild red New Mexican chile powder, or to taste
1 dried chipotle pepper, crumbled
1 tablespoon dried whole oregano
1 tablespoon ground cumin
1/2 teaspoon allspice
1 large can (28 ounces) crushed tomatoes
5 cloves garlic, mashed
salt to taste

GARNISHES
1 chopped raw onion
2 chopped tomatoes
2 cups shredded lettuce
1 dozen tortillas

1. Pick over the beans to remove foreign objects, wash, and soak in water overnight. Drain.

2. Cover beans with fresh water to cover by 2 inches, bring to a boil, lower heat, partially cover, and cook until tender, about 2 hours, keeping water level constant by adding water as needed.

3. Meanwhile, sauté the onions in the olive oil over medium heat until golden. Add the chile powder, chipotle pepper, oregano, cumin, and allspice. Cook together for 2 minutes.

4. Add the tomatoes and simmer for 5 minutes.

5. Add this mixture to beans along with the garlic. Simmer the beans, partially covered, for another hour or so, being careful not

to let them burn, until they become creamy and start to melt into the liquid.

6. Add salt to taste and more chile if you want a hotter dish. Serve in bowls with garnishes: chopped raw onion, chopped tomatoes, shredded lettuce, warm tortillas.

You can vary the chili by adding any of the following items along with the tomato-and-onion mixture: fresh shiitake or other mushrooms, sautéed in olive oil until beginning to brown (or use reconstituted dried mushrooms), sliced carrots, or wheat meat (wheat gluten, available in dried form at natural-food stores). Also experiment with dashes of balsamic vinegar.

❧ *Barley Salad* ❧

3 cups vegetable stock (see pages 89–91) or water
1 cup pearl barley
salt to taste

DRESSING
3 tablespoons olive oil
3 tablespoons fresh lemon juice
3–4 cloves garlic, mashed
salt to taste

1/2 cup chopped fresh parsley
1 bunch scallions, sliced thin
1 bunch radishes, sliced
1 cucumber, peeled, seeded, and diced
1 red bell pepper, seeded and sliced
1/2 cup chopped fresh mint

1. Bring to a boil the vegetable stock (or water). Add barley and salt if desired. Cover, reduce heat, and simmer until barley is tender and liquid is absorbed, about 45 minutes.

2. Mix the dressing and pour it over barley.

3. Allow barley to cool, then add the parsley, scallions, radishes, cucumber, red pepper, and mint. (If you do not have fresh mint, add 1/4 cup dried spearmint to the dressing.)

4. Mix well and chill for several hours before serving.

✌ *Asian Coleslaw* ✌

1 medium head green cabbage
1 medium head red cabbage
3 tablespoons sea salt
3 large carrots

DRESSING
2/3 cup unseasoned rice vinegar
1/4 cup light-brown sugar
1 1/2 tablespoons dark-roasted sesame oil

minced scallions and toasted sesame seeds (optional)

1. Discard outer leaves of cabbages. Cut heads in quarters; remove and discard cores. Slice cabbage thinly or shred in a food
processor. Place it in a large bowl in batches and sprinkle the sea
salt over it. Toss to distribute salt evenly and let cabbage sit for 1
hour to soften.

2. Meanwhile, peel the carrots and grate them into thin shreds.

3. Drain off any liquid produced by cabbage and wash cabbage
well in cold water to remove excess salt. Taste the cabbage; if it is
still too salty, wash again.

4. Add carrots and dressing. Mix well, correct seasoning, and let
chill for at least an hour before serving. Optional additions: minced
scallions and toasted sesame seeds.

Serves 8.

✌ *Festive Wild Rice* ✌

1 cup dried mushrooms
1 cup wild rice
1/2 cup freshly squeezed orange juice
1/4 cup dry sherry
1/2 cup sliced carrots
2 tablespoons chopped fresh parsley
salt or natural soy sauce to taste
1/3 cup finely chopped black walnuts, pecans, or filberts (optional)

1. Soak the dried mushrooms in water to cover until they are soft. Squeeze them out, reserving liquid, and slice.

2. Wash the wild rice well in cold water and place in pot with the mushroom-soaking liquid (minus any sediment) and enough additional cold water to total 2 cups.

3. Add the orange juice, sherry, and carrots. Bring to a boil, reduce heat, cover, and simmer for 30 minutes.

4. Add mushrooms and continue cooking until rice is tender and all the liquid is absorbed.

5. Add the chopped parsley and salt or natural soy sauce to taste. Optional: stir in 1/3 cup finely chopped nuts (black walnuts, pecans, or filberts).

⤜ *Tofu with Cilantro Sauce* ⤛

1-pound cake firm tofu
1 tablespoon salt

SAUCE
1 tablespoon canola oil
1 tablespoon finely chopped fresh gingerroot
1/2 cup chopped fresh cilantro
1 tablespoon natural soy sauce
1 teaspoon light-brown sugar

1. Cut the tofu into 4 thick slices. Place slices in a pot containing 3 cups cold water and the salt. Soak for 30 minutes, then slowly bring it almost to a boil, and cook without boiling for 5 minutes.

2. While tofu is heating, prepare the sauce. Heat the canola oil in a skillet and add the ginger. Stir-fry for 1 minute, then add the cilantro, soy sauce, and sugar. Cook for 1 minute over high heat.

3. Remove tofu from heat, drain, carefully transfer to a warm serving dish, and spoon sauce over it.

Mental/Spiritual

Your assignment here is not unrelated to the project assignment for this week. I am asking you to reach out and resume connection with someone from whom you are estranged—in other words, to practice forgiveness.

Human relationships are complex, often marked by upheavals. The joy of intimate connection is often balanced by the pain of separation and estrangement. When people who have been close separate, there is usually a great deal of hurt and blame, since each party feels wronged and justified in maintaining distance. To take the first step toward reconciliation is difficult, requiring emotional maturity and skill; it can also put you more in contact with your higher self. To err is human, to forgive divine.

If you can start the process of healing a damaged relationship this week, you will have my great respect. Regardless of the outcome, you will have demonstrated a willingness to repair a connection that was once important to you, and that willingness in itself is healthy. If you succeed, you will have regained a lost friend. If you do not succeed, you will still have improved your well-being, because forgiveness benefits oneself, not just another. By forgiving, you can lessen your own emotional pain and experience increased inner peace, no matter what the response of the other person. It is possible to practice forgiveness toward persons who are unreachable or even deceased, because you still carry them in your memory and your heart and can enter into an inner dialogue with them.

In his book *Healing into Life and Death,* Stephen Levine gives a forgiveness meditation that can be used in this way. I am going to quote part of it as an example of how you can forgive someone inwardly even if external communication is not possible.

Begin by slowly bringing into your mind, into your heart, the image of someone for whom you have some resentment. Gently allow a picture, a feeling, a sense of them to gather there. Gently now invite them into your heart just for this moment.

Notice whatever fear or anger may arise to limit or deny their entrance and soften gently all about it. No force. Just an experiment in truth which invites this person in.

And silently in your heart say to this person, "I forgive you."

Open to a sense of their presence and say, "I forgive you for whatever pain you may have caused me in the past, intentionally or unintentionally, through your words, your thoughts, your actions. However you may have caused me pain in the past, I forgive you."

Feel for even a moment the spaciousness of relating to that person with the possibility of forgiveness.

Let go of those walls, those curtains of resentment, so that your heart may be free. So that your life may be lighter.

"I forgive you for whatever you may have done that caused me pain, intentionally or unintentionally, through your actions, through your words, even through your thoughts, through whatever you did. Through whatever you didn't do. However the pain came to me through you, I forgive you. I forgive you."

Of course, if you decide to try this meditation, you should do it with full attention and concentration, and no distractions. Feel free to change the wording to suit your own style and needs, and notice how you feel afterward.

The tasks that I have given you this week are somewhat different from those of the six previous weeks, and I expect that some readers will have difficulty with them. Doing service work and practicing forgiveness may not be as easy as taking vitamin C or trying a dish of kale, but they are central elements of this Eight-Week Program. Healing relationships, emotional pain, and the sense of isolation that is at the root of much human disease is a necessary step in helping the healing system perform most efficiently. A program for optimum health that omitted this kind of work would be incomplete.

Optional

If you would like to continue experimenting with dietary restriction, try limiting your intake one day this week to fruit juice, water, and herbal tea. Again, freshly made juice is best, if you can get it; otherwise use natural juice without added sugar. Some bottled fruit juice may give you very concentrated sweetness, and you may wish to dilute it with water. This will prepare you to try a water fast next week, if you are so inclined.

A Healing Story:
The Power of Intimacy

Peter R., a forty-year-old writer in New York, married with children, sends me this account:

> I'm going to tell you my story of sex, intimacy, and curing the com-
> mon cold simply because it describes one of the most astounding
> things that have ever happened to me.
>
> I was an eighteen-year-old freshman in college, totally and com-
> pletely in love with my girlfriend. It was an all-encompassing, full-
> force, mind-body-and-soul kind of thing. My healing took place on
> a winter evening, a Friday night, when I was in the third or fourth
> day of what promised to be a miserable nine-day cold (three days
> getting sick, three being sick, three getting well). I had all the symp-
> toms: sore throat, stuffed nose, fever, fatigue. I hadn't gone to
> classes that day and hadn't heard from my girlfriend, so I assumed
> that she'd made other plans for the evening. Obviously, I was too
> sick to go out or entertain her in any way.
>
> She showed up at about six. I imagine that I pulled on a pair of
> jeans when I heard her knock on the door. I probably hadn't
> shaved, showered, or combed my hair for a few days and must have
> looked wretched but couldn't have cared less. I must have been
> happy to see her—I always was—but I know I was astonished and
> touched when this young woman, who was no Florence Nightin-
> gale, gave me a big, fat, open-mouthed, romantic kiss on the mouth
> and proceeded to undress. I remember being so moved by her want-
> ing to be intimate with me on that particular night. You see, I come

from the school where you pretty much keep your germs to yourself, staying away from people when you're sick. And here was this girl, the love of my young life, who was willing to catch a cold, to ignore her own health in order to be with me, to make love with me. Which is what we did until dawn. Then we slept.

When I awoke, probably late the next morning, I swear that the sore throat, stuffy nose, fever—all of it—was gone. Something about the intensity of the intimacy and sex burned the thing right out of me. No drugs, no nothing but touch, taste, sound, smell, and two hearts coming together as one. It was much, much more effective than "Take two pills and call me in the morning."

12

WEEK EIGHT

Projects

• Review the changes you have made in your lifestyle in the program so far and think about how many of them you wish to make permanent. Develop a realistic plan that you can stick to over the next eight weeks.

Diet

• Think about how you can continue the dietary changes of this program in coming weeks.

Supplements

• Start taking your tonic. Make a commitment to give it a two-month trial to see what it does for your energy level, resistance, and outlook.

Exercise

• Reach your goal of a forty-five-minute walk, five days of the week.

Mental/Spiritual

• Continue the breathing exercises. Start using the Relaxing Breath whenever you feel anxious or upset, and be sure to do it at least twice a day.

• Maintain your news fast for the whole week. At the end of the week, think about how much news you want to let back into your life in coming weeks.

• Think of people who have hurt you or made you angry. Try to bring yourself to understand their actions and forgive them. Can you express forgiveness to at least one of them?

• Reward yourself with especially beautiful flowers for completing this program. Why not also buy flowers for someone else?

Optional

• Try a one-day water fast this week. You can have herbal tea with lemon if you like, but nothing caloric. If this proves too difficult, drink some diluted fruit juice. Take vitamin C but skip the other supplements this day.

COMMENTARY

Congratulations! You have almost made it to the end of the Eight-Week Program. This week you will be fine-tuning the adjustments of previous weeks and getting ready to solidify a new, healthier lifestyle that will serve you for the rest of your life. I am sure you realize by now that this program is not an eight-week diet or crash fitness plan that you can abandon once you have achieved a limited goal—like looking good in a new bathing suit. Following all the instructions and then going back to your old ways of living is not the point. Continuing to move in the direction of optimum health is.

Projects

I would like you to start thinking about Week Nine. Are you going to be able to stick with the many changes that I have asked you to make in your life so far? Are any unrealistic for you? (Maybe by now you have decided that you really hate broccoli.)

The question this week is how you can carry this plan forward. If it is going to work for you, it has to suit you and be adaptable to the particular circumstances of your life. In the next section of the book, I present a number of customized plans for people with special needs: the young, the old, pregnant women, those with particular disease risks. I suggest that you look over all of this information to get a sense of how the program can be modified; please understand that it is very flexible in its details. I want you to adhere to the spirit of the program, to its essence, and modify the details so that they work for you without being a burden or making you feel deprived or constrained. Improved health should bring with it a sense of greater freedom, joy, and lightness of being.

Please review with me the projects of past weeks and consider how you can advance them into Week Nine and beyond.

In Week One, I asked you to become aware of unhealthy items in your stock of foods. I do not see much difficulty here. Once you understand the impact that certain fats, artificial sweeteners, and artificial colors have on your body's healing potential, you should find it easy to exclude them from your home. If you eat a lot of meat and dairy products, you will have to cut down on them because of their content of saturated fat. Remember that cheese is the major source of saturated fat in the Western diet, and start there. The recommendation throughout the Eight-Week Program to cut down on animal foods is totally in line with current medical and scientific thinking about reducing the risks of diseases that kill and disable people prematurely in our society. As I write, the American Cancer Society has just released new dietary guidelines that urge cutting consumption of high-fat foods, particularly those from animal sources. "Use meat as a side dish," the society says, "rather than as the focus of a meal."

I do not think you will find it hard to learn to rely on good olive oil as your main oil in food preparation, but one difficulty you will face is avoiding products made with partially hydrogenated fats, since these are ubiquitous. You must get in the habit of reading labels and go to the trouble of finding alternative products, possibly in natural-food stores.

In Week Two, I asked you to think about your drinking water and take the necessary steps to ensure its purity. That entailed some homework and perhaps some expenditure, but once you take the necessary action, there are no further demands. I do not want you to be paranoid about water you encounter when you are away from home. I do want you to reduce long-term exposure to water-borne toxins that can compromise your body's healing system.

The main project of Week Three—learning about organic produce—required both homework and an ongoing commitment. You will certainly have to go to extra trouble and expense to obtain chemical-free fruits and vegetables, but you can make your task easier by learning the most contaminated crops and adjusting your purchases accordingly. There is no value in worrying about the nonorganic produce that you eat; concentrate instead on trying to follow this recommendation to whatever extent you can, knowing that you will be helping your body reduce its toxic load. I also want to remind you that, however you can help increase demand for fruits and vegetables grown without agrichemicals, you will be making the job easier for all of us in the future, because organic agriculture is following consumer demand; as it spreads, the quality and availability of organic produce will increase, and prices will come down.

The other project this week was to remove or distance yourself from sources of toxic energy. That meant some inconvenience, perhaps, but I do not think it is a difficult recommendation to follow.

In much the same way, the projects of Week Four require one-time effort and expense: correcting impediments to good sleep, and improving air quality in your home with filters or house plants.

In Week Five, I asked you to experiment with sweat bathing in a sauna or steam room. Now that you are finishing the program, you can decide how often you want to continue this practice. If you like it, I recommend it as an ongoing addition to your lifestyle at whatever frequency is convenient. Perhaps you have located a facility you can use at a nearby health or fitness club or a friend's house. If you can see benefits for you, you might consider installing a sauna or steam room in your own home. When I moved to a new house three years ago, I had an old closet converted to a steam room that my wife and I use regularly except in the Arizona summer. Relatively inexpensive steam units are available for installation into a bath enclosure. If you find all of this too much trouble and not enough to your liking, you can just take the occasional steam or sauna when you have overindulged in food or drink, been in contact with toxins, or feel that your healing system could use a boost.

The Week Six project was to inform yourself about tonics and to locate a product that you could start using now. Begin to take your tonic regularly this week, and keep doing so for a full two months. At the end of that time, make an assessment of what it appears to be doing for you and decide whether you want to continue. Remember that the tonics I described are nontoxic and can be used over long periods of time; in fact, their benefits often appear gradually and accrue cumulatively only after long-term, regular use.

Finally, last week I asked you to do some service work, to put the needs and interests of others ahead of your own in some way of your choosing. Of course, I did not intend this suggestion to expire at the end of the week. As I have explained, the practice of giving some of your time and energy to help others without any expectation of return will, in fact, bring you great returns in improved spiritual, mental, and, eventually, physical health, if it becomes an ongoing part of your life. I will leave it to you to figure out how you can implement this project and keep it going. Maybe you do something of the sort already and just need to recognize it for what it is. Maybe you have to develop it a bit. It's up to you.

Diet

All dietary changes are hard, but I think the ones I have suggested here are not that wrenching and might actually show you new ways to experience pleasure in eating; besides, you can enjoy knowing that you are giving your body nutrients it can use to protect and enhance its healing ability. Let me review these changes with you in order to identify any obstacles to your continuing with them after this week.

The recommendations of Week One—to add broccoli and salmon or sardines to your diet—should not be difficult. If you do not care for sardines and do not want to cook salmon at home, it is very easy to get it in restaurants, for it seems now to be a regular menu choice everywhere. Remember that medical researchers strongly recommend eating more fish in place of meat. Remember also that you can always use flaxseeds as an alternative source of omega-3 fatty acids if you do not like fish. Increasing intake of omega-3s as part of your regular diet is a form of health insurance as you grow older, since these compounds aid the body in ways that reduce risks of many diseases.

As for broccoli, if you do hate it by now, note that the general recommendation here is to eat more fresh fruits and vegetables; broccoli is just representative of that category of foods, and if you really do not like it, you have many other choices (including its cruciferous relatives: cabbage, kale, and cauliflower). I will acknowledge that the preparation of fresh vegetables takes some skill and time. For that reason, I have given you easy and delicious recipes that I hope will give you ideas for other dishes. The master broccoli recipe takes about ten minutes from start to finish, easily worth it in terms of the goodness of the result and its contribution to health. Cleaning and chopping vegetables can be relaxing, a kind of meditation that helps you let go of the worries of the day. If, for convenience, you must eat frozen vegetables, do so; they are certainly better than no vegetables. Or make a point of eating vegetables when you dine out.

In Week Two I asked you to eat more whole-grain products as well as to approach soybeans. The first recommendation should not be hard to continue unless you are a real white-flour junkie. Even so, you can add some whole-grain dishes to your diet. As for soy foods, I hope that since Week Three you have found some that you will want to keep on eating, or that you have learned to like some of the tofu and tempeh recipes I provided. Soy foods make it possible to cut back further on meat and still enjoy the flavors and textures of animal foods. Since this will be a stretch for some of you, I can only encourage you to keep experimenting until you find soy products you like. Really, they are out there, and if you will make them part of your diet, they will give you a wonderful nutritional nudge in the direction of better long-term health.

Also in Week Two, I asked you to give green tea a try, particularly if you use other forms of caffeine. Note that I am not telling you to give up coffee. (You can read elsewhere what I have written about the effects of that beverage on health.) I just want you to try something new and consider adding it as a tonic, or using it to replace some of your other sources of caffeine.

I can't imagine that you will have trouble keeping garlic in your life, even if it was not there to begin with. Its health benefits are so numerous and well documented and its flavor so appealing in so many different kinds of food that I cannot believe this suggestion from Week Four would present any difficulty, except to those who must get over unfounded fears of offending others by smelling of this wonderful herb. It should be just as easy for you to continue eating more ginger, which you started to do in Week Five.

Adding cooked greens to your diet, as I asked you to do in Week Six, may be harder, both because these vegetables may be new to you and because it takes some effort to cook them. I hope you will rely on the recipes here, because I've developed them to show you the versatility of greens and their relative ease of preparation. I can turn a bunch of kale into a delicious main dish in about fifteen minutes, and I have confidence that you can too. Greens are cheap and highly nutritious. Once you get to know them and see the possibilities for using them, I think it will be easier for you to eat them often.

And that is the sum total of the dietary changes the program asked you to make—not so burdensome, I think, that you should not be able to keep them going into Week Nine and beyond.

Supplements

All you have to do here is remember to take your antioxidant formula every day. That means having a daily routine for taking the three vitamins and selenium and making sure you do not run out of any of them. You can and should take them for the rest of your life. The benefits in terms of reduced disease risks are too great to pass up.

Exercise

Your challenge here will be time. Can you find the time for a brisk forty-five-minute walk most days of the week? Maybe you are lucky enough to be able to walk to work or walk partway to work. Maybe you will have to spend some time on a treadmill in a fitness club. (I do not like that as much as real walking, but it serves some people well.) Maybe you can do your walking in a mall while shopping. The point here is to use your body in ways that are sensible and nontraumatic. If you already have an exercise regimen that you are happy with, stick with it, and try also to do some walking. Remember that walking offers health benefits that other forms of exercise may not, and that it will continue to serve you as a best exercise into old age. Do it whenever you can, as much as you find comfortable and congruent with your lifestyle.

Stretching should be easier for you, since it takes little time and feels so good. Whether or not you decide to practice yoga or some other formal system, remember the general principle: whenever your body has been in one position for a time, give it a stretch in the opposite direction.

Mental/Spiritual

The prescriptions I gave you under this heading are the most distinctive elements of the Eight-Week Program, and they are absolutely essential to it. Many experts who promote healthy living give lip service to the role of mental and spiritual factors in shaping total health, but few are able to provide concrete, practical advice about working with them. I have given you a number of exercises and assignments here that I hope you have found interesting and worthwhile enough so you want to incorporate them into your life on an ongoing basis.

The breathing exercises are critical. Taking very little time and effort, they give immediate rewards and immeasurable long-term benefits, so please stick with them. If you enjoy observing your breath, experiment with extending the time that you devote to it, since this is a painless, gentle way of developing a meditation practice. I have come to believe that breath is the master key to optimum health, both because of its direct effects on physiology, especially of the nervous system, and because it is the ultimate link that joins body, mind, and spirit. No other component of the Eight-Week Program has such potential to improve your well-being for such a small investment of time and effort.

If my recommendations to enjoy flowers, parks, music, and art give you trouble, you are beyond my help. The more you allow these influences into your life, the happier and healthier you will be.

This week I have asked you to try to exclude news from your life for seven full days, a really serious news fast. Remember: I do not want you to be uninformed about the state of the world. I do want you to discover and make use of the fact that you have choice as to how much news you allow into your consciousness, especially if it disturbs your emotional and spiritual equilibrium. Beginning in Week Nine, you can decide how much of it to let back in.

I also want you to bring the concept of healing more into your awareness from now on. Continue to note your own experiences of it, inquire about the experiences of others, read about healing, discuss it with family, friends, and colleagues, even perhaps with your doctor. The simple and—I think—self-evident ideas that the body can heal itself if given a chance, that it wants to be healthy, and that the tremendous healing power of nature is always there to help are missing from contemporary medical research, teaching, and practice. The more we can bring them back into intellectual discourse in our society, the sooner medical research, teaching, and practice will begin to embrace them again. That change would benefit all of us, because, as I have written over the years, the way we experience reality is influenced by the concepts we have or do not have in our heads. The more we focus on healing as an everyday event, the more it will happen for us.

Finally, I have asked you to do some work in the area of human relations: to seek out and spend more time with people who raise your spirits, to try to heal damaged relationships, and to practice compassion and forgiveness by trying to understand the actions of others and forgiving them, either internally or externally. These are all general recommendations that do not require you to adhere to any particular regimen or schedule. Rather, they indicate a direction of importance in optimizing health, because the quality of our interactions with our fellow humans is powerfully influential on our own states of body, mind, and spirit. Obviously, this is ongoing work that should simply become part of the way you live. It requires nothing more than recognition of the importance of human relations and a willingness to try to improve your own.

Optional

If you have followed the optional suggestions in recent weeks, try a true fast one day this week: nothing but water and herbal tea. Do not expect to have boundless energy, or even enough to do your usual routines. You might do this on the weekend, when you can take it easy and keep yourself amused and comfortable despite not eating. Stay warm—some people get cold when they do not stoke the metabolic furnace—and do not make it harder on yourself by keeping other people company while they eat. Pay attention to how you feel, and how the experience of eating is different when you break your fast the next morning.

If these experiments have agreed with you, consider repeating them in the future—if you feel you are catching a cold, for example, or want to give your digestive system a rest following a period of overeating, or want to continue to explore the effects of dietary restriction and fasting on consciousness.

Once again, it is a pleasure to congratulate you on completing this program. I know that it will continue to work for you in the coming weeks and years.

In the following pages, I present a number of healing stories from people who followed the Eight-Week Program. Note that they used common sense, were flexible, and modified the recommendations to suit their own particular needs.

A Healing Story:
A Couple Follows the Program

Roy and Marybeth Dawson of Tucson, Arizona, describe their experiences as follows:

We began your program in August 1995.

Week One: Out with the margarine, in with the olive oil. Always have eaten broccoli. Didn't eat salmon, sardines, or kippers; never got around to flaxseed. Increased vitamin-C dosage. Already walked two miles (fifteen minutes a mile) daily. (Roy had uneventful recovery from a prostatectomy two years ago—lots of positive thinking throughout.) Need more work on Breath Observation. Our cats eat the fresh flowers; we will have to observe flowers from afar.

Week Two: I drank bottled water; Roy continued drinking from the tap. Bought soy burgers and green tea (good!). We ate lots of carrots, didn't take beta-carotene. Our house in the country gives us "beauty overload"—no need for parks. News fasts are easy (we do watch the weather).

Week Three: No organic produce nearby, but we buy fresh produce at local farm markets. Moved clock radio away from nightstand. I take vitamin E; Roy can't—he's on Coumadin [a prescription anticoagulant].

Week Four: Sleeping area is restful. Need to eat more garlic. Have cut way back on meat to once a week or less. Need to remember to do breathing exercises. Still walking two fifteen-minute miles daily.

Week Five: Steam bath/sauna not available. Bought crystallized ginger. We listen to beautiful music almost daily.

Week Six: Our tonic is a commercial product that is a mixture of herbs with honey, molasses, bee pollen, vitamins, and minerals. We take it every day.

Week Seven: Service work has included volunteering at Sabino Canyon [park], leading nature hikes and getting people enthused about the out-of-doors, nature's "tonic." We do it whenever possible. Our walk remains at two miles, thirty minutes daily.

Week Eight: We will continue as above.

Results: Subtle effects include a more positive attitude, mental patterns are calmer, more relaxed. Physical symptoms have lessened or disappeared. For example, Roy's tennis elbow, which was treated unsuccessfully with cortisone, is completely healed. Also psoriasis on the palms—almost 100 percent improvement. I had a drop in cholesterol from 205 to 183 along with an increase in HDL and a decrease in blood pressure.

The most profound effect is in general resistance. We both have worked in the resort business for ten years and have a great deal of contact with travelers and germs. We had got used to annual bouts of sickness requiring antibiotics. Since we started the program we have not had a single day of illness.

We've just completed building a straw-bale house and came through the experience unscathed, physically and mentally. We are building a sweat lodge for our steam baths and are continuing to incorporate in our daily lives what we have learned from the program. Thanks!

A Healing Story:
Mind over Back Pain

THIS REPORT COMES from Edie Crawford of Camp Verde, Arizona:

Last summer (1995), while we were driving from Arizona to the Adirondacks in New York, I read about the Eight-Week Program, and started it on arrival at our destination. I loved the idea of buying flowers weekly and had a wonderful time going to the florist. In Arizona I live in the wilderness and enjoy wildflowers but can't actually get to a florist; this was a source of much pleasure. I also thoroughly enjoyed the breathing exercises and still do them. I eat flaxseeds pretty regularly, added to yogurt for lunch. I did already take vitamin C, so I added vitamin E, selenium, carotene, calcium, and magnesium, and I walked daily. (I was suffering chronic back pain and "couldn't" do much else. Happily, I read the book you recommended [*Healing Back Pain: The Mind-Body Connection* by John Sarno, M.D. (New York: Warner, 1991)], understood the nature of the problem, and began to play tennis, run, sail, swim, windsurf, canoe, return to Arizona to row the Grand Canyon, and ride.

I have adopted soy milk for breakfast with cereal. I already observed a news fast and only sporadically catch up with a paper or radio, but it was wonderful to have my instinct for this affirmed.

I drink more ginger tea and eat garlic regularly. We built a sweat lodge at our ranch. I try to eat more broccoli and fish.

I find I can let go of hurt much faster and forgive. There have been a lot of hurt feelings among members of my family, and all this has helped.

I also did some guided imagery that summer, which I learned from a book. I still meditate, walk, and do yoga daily except when traveling or running Grand Canyon trips.

A Healing Story:
Report from Michigan

THIS REPORT DESCRIBES Julia Sermersheim's experience with the program. She lives in Battle Creek, Michigan.

I have followed about 90 percent of your ideas over the past three and a half years, not just for eight weeks.

I cleaned out my pantry and use mainly olive oil and a little butter. I eat broccoli weekly and some salmon and flaxseed oil. I take one gram of vitamin C after each meal. Walking is a problem: I get fatigued if I walk more than twenty minutes two times a week.

I drink distilled water and use it in herbal teas. Just completed a macrobiotic-cooking class and am eating more beans, grains, fruits, veggies, and sea vegetables. I drink green tea. Am taking beta-carotene in a multivitamin supplement.

Mainly I buy organic beans and grains. I don't have an electric blanket, nor a TV, VCR, or computer, and I stopped using the microwave. For breakfast I eat only fruit. I eat less meat and more beans and grains. I take vitamin E and selenium. I like to read books about mind/body medicine, acupuncture and acupressure, and about creative people. My creative outlet is making fabric wall pieces.

My bedroom is very quiet, and I do not heat it in the winter. The fresh air is wonderful and smells cleaner and fresher than in the rest of the house. I eat lots of garlic (three to four cloves two or three times a week). I work part-time.

I have not done a steam bath but plan to. I look forward to trying ginger tea and doing more walking.

I have taken milk thistle. My acupuncturist told me not to take ginseng—it heats my body too much. I've been experimenting with other nutritional supplements and have seen a new level of energy and endurance evolve. Just went to see the Degas exhibit in Chicago—wonderful.

I do volunteer work at various organizations. Through seminars and courses, I've been learning how to put the past in the past and to live more in the present, and how to resolve estranged relationships. I am also attending church regularly and enjoy the members there. I can express forgiveness to people who have hurt me. I have enjoyed the flowers in my garden, especially the rosebush my father gave to my mother more than thirty years ago. They have both died, and I cherish the beautiful roses that the bush still produces every year.

A Healing Story: K.G.'s Adventure

THE LAWYER who wrote this account asked that I not use her name, so I will identify her only as Mrs. K.G.:

I had copies of your books, but I believed myself to be too busy and too tired from work and caring for my four children (youngest seven, oldest twelve) to take the time to read them—that is, until I had two serious reactions to prescribed medicines within a span of ten months. The first was caused by a too-high dose of a form of ergotamine, an injected drug for migraines. By the time I got the headache specialist to believe that I was in trouble, there was no detectable pulse in my lower arms and legs. I was in indescribable pain that morphine did not touch. I spent three days in September 1994 in an intensive-care unit under the care of toxicologists. The second episode was an allergic reaction to a sulfa drug in July 1995. I couldn't stand the idea of another hospitalization, so I stayed at home and watched my skin "boil." I sat in tubs of ice water and swallowed most of a new prescription of asthma medication to keep me breathing. I know I'm lucky to be alive.

A neurologist I consulted on the advice of the toxicologists eventually came to the conclusion that I should learn to deal with my migraines without drugs and sent me to a wonderful holistic medical doctor. That doctor identified a number of things I would have to "fix" before I could feel really well again. I was most concerned with having a strategy I could use right away for coping with migraines, so he told me to practice the breathing exercises in your books. And that is how I came to learn of the Eight-Week Program.

In Week One I started using extra-virgin olive oil. I did not clean out my pantry, because I'm not a good enough cook to understand substitutions, but I did buy a healthy-foods cookbook. I ate broccoli and took vitamin C, started walking, and did all the mental/spiritual exercises except bringing flowers home (allergies). Instead, I tried to make a point of noticing nature.

In Week Two I bought organic foods at local markets, checked on my bottled water to be sure it was OK, ate fish, drank some green tea (yuck! but then I'm not a coffee or tea drinker anyway), and added a carotene supplement. I also increased my walking. I had trouble remembering to do the breathing exercises regularly. I enjoyed having a justification for limiting my intake of news.

In Week Three I concentrated on fruits and vegetables and fish but found I did not take to soy products (allergies). I do not have an electric blanket, and I do not use a computer. The clock radio has not left my husband's nightstand and is not likely to, ever. I started reading inspirational books suggested by my physician. I called a law-school classmate I hadn't seen in years and we had lunch. I also sent flowers to a friend.

In Week Four I paid attention to my sleeping area and got air filters for the kids' rooms. Tried garlic but really didn't stick with it. I also reduced my intake of animal protein, enjoyed limited news fasts, and read articles about healing. Though I still couldn't remember to do the breathing regularly, I did eventually learn to try relaxation breathing when I felt a headache coming.

In Week Five I invented my own steam bath—I sat in a hot garage with the dryer running with a load of towels—a very steamy and hot experience. Tried crystallized ginger, and I loved it. I increased the walking further—easier since I've been stretching and getting osteopathic treatments. I never made it past two days of news fasting; my job requires a certain amount of awareness of local and national events. Still, I make a point of avoiding articles about hurt children or animals and never listen to network news. I bought a tape of meditation music and carry it everywhere. I use it in stressful situations: traffic jams, dentist office, long car trips.

In Week Six I decided to use astragalus as a tonic. I'm still on it. I gave up the steam bath but stuck with everything else.

In Weeks Seven and Eight I kept up the walking, the appreciation of art, music, and nature, the supplements and herbs, the fish, fruits and vegetables, and my reading. I experimented with herbs and vitamins suggested in your books for various complaints.

Since then I continue to practice many of the things I learned from the Eight-Week Program. I am also studying yoga and still trying to learn healthier recipes. I'm giving up the practice of law because its rewards do not make up for the wear and tear on me. (I was amazed when I recalled that you had said in your books that just such a change might be necessary.)

So far I can say for myself that I look and feel much better, and I am much happier than I've been since college days. With a little more effort I can improve even further. I have more energy. I am interested in learning all sorts of new things. I feel so good now as a result of osteopathic treatment, acupuncture, massage, and stretching that I can dance again, one of my chief delights. I'm reading purely for fun again (haven't done much of that since college). My marriage is vastly improved—my husband of twenty-two years says it's because I'm nicer when I feel better. I have far fewer migraines, and I take much less medicine. I plan to learn to do the breathing exercises regularly and have no doubt I will discover many rewards from making them a part of my life.

13

Week Nine and Beyond

Projects

• Stick with the program.

Diet

• Include:
  Broccoli
  Fish or flax
  Fruits and vegetables, organic when possible
  Soy foods
  Whole grains
  Cooked greens
  Garlic and ginger
• And enjoy!

Supplements

• Continue with your antioxidants.

Exercise

• Walk.
• Stretch.

Mental/Spiritual

- Breathe.
- Flowers, nature, music, art.
- Choose your news carefully.
- Think about healing.
- Forgiveness.

In the following pages, I present a few more examples of people who followed the program and made real changes in their lives. It can make a real change in your life too!

A Healing Story:
Selected Elements
of the Program

Eleanor Engelhardt, a licensed massage therapist from Youngstown, Ohio, tells me she has used parts of the program:

I have olive or canola oil, fresh broccoli, collards or other greens every day. I put flaxseeds over my cereal and eat flaxseed/sunflower-seed bread. I take vitamin C with each meal, as well as the other antioxidants. I eat whole grains and vegetables and drink filtered water. I follow a vegan diet.

The walking each day is so important to mental and spiritual health. I also do yoga and ride a bike. I keep a diary to weed out negative thinking patterns. I take time in parks, where I read, walk, and do Breath Observation. I also do daily light-and-sound meditations.

I recommend all of this to clients and students, along with a reading list of spiritual books.

A Healing Story:
Report from a Lady Barber

Margo Murdock of Macon, Georgia, is not only a barber but also an adventurous traveler, and a health counselor to her clients. She says that, when you've got someone in the chair and a razor in your hand, you've got the person's full attention. Margo writes:

I could be the poster child for your work, since I've followed your advice for years—sixteen, to be exact. Goldenseal and comfrey have saved me bunches. I tried to slice off the tip of my little finger with a straight razor a while back. I cleaned it with hydrogen peroxide, put goldenseal on it and a butterfly closure. Next day I cleaned it again with peroxide and covered it with comfrey: no infection, no scar, no nothing.

Last year, in Nepal, I put a piece of bamboo basket through my arm. I used bottled water, goldenseal, and comfrey: no infection, no scar, no nothing. I use nettles for allergies, mullein oil for my granddaughters' ears. I've tried all of your natural remedies, and everything works.

As for the program: I use only olive and canola oils. I'm allergic to fish, so can't do it. Instead I use a cereal with flaxseeds. I take the antioxidant formula. I do the breathing exercises religiously and teach them to my clients. I serve only distilled water at home and in my shop. I'm not crazy about green tea but drink it some. I buy only organic (when I cook).

I love the news fast. (I used to be addicted to television news.)

I moved all the electrical stuff away from my bed and got an air filter for the bedroom. It made a *huge difference.* (I have cats.)

I took a trip alone with my mother (we both survived), became a grandmother for the second time, and started my own shop. I took a course in seated (chair) massage and went to "spiritual boot camp."

My energy level is good, my attitude great. How's that for a program that works? It's kept me healthy!

A HEALING STORY:
A PATIENT WITH MULTIPLE SCLEROSIS

JOYCE DOOLEY of Ridgecrest, California, sent me this report:

The Eight-Week Program has changed my life totally! I followed as much of it as I safely could without jeopardizing my health. I have multiple sclerosis, the kind that relapses and remits.

I promptly started using extra-virgin olive oil. I had already decided to become a vegetarian, and the program helped immensely. Like you, I love broccoli and eat it several times weekly. I eat fish sources of omega-3 fatty acids occasionally but eat tofu almost every day. I ingest many supplements—vitamin C, a multivitamin, folic acid, potassium, magnesium, and calcium on a daily basis. I tried 200 IU of vitamin E, then 400, then went up to 800, but found that amount caused my usually normal blood pressure to rise, so I stopped it.

Garlic has become a favorite, as has ginger. Fruits and vegetables are staples in my diet. I avoid the news as much as possible these days. I practice breathing exercises and have come up with my own form of imagery/visualization.

I've used, when necessary, dong quai, chaste tree, maitake, and echinacea. I do not choose to go on a fast of any type, as I'm very thin, and my appetite fluctuates as it is. And as I am supposed to avoid the heat, I do not desire to use a steam bath or sauna.

Last but by *no* means least, I walk. I quickly went from ten minutes for five days of the week to forty-five minutes or more, at least five days of the week and usually every day, at a very brisk pace.

Since I should not overheat, I have to be careful. On hot days I can walk inside on a treadmill with the air conditioner revved up, a glass of iced water available, and a fan blowing on me, which allow me to continue my very favorite exercise. I live in the Mojave Desert, and in the extreme heat, I sometimes take one or two buffered aspirin to cool my body core before walking.

A Healing Story:
Peripheral Neuropathy

This account comes from Arline Birdwell Phelps of Muleshoe, Texas:

In November 1995, I was diagnosed with peripheral neuropathy. I could only walk with a cane and was miserable! My doctor advised a severe drug treatment to suppress my immune system. This idea was so frightening to me that I stopped being her patient and did nothing until my son gave me your book. After following the Eight-Week Program, I continued the diet, vitamin, and exercise routines. By mid-April, I was walking without my cane, could go to a furniture market in North Carolina, and continue to take care of my business.

I grew up on a diet high in protein and low in complex carbohydrates, with no food supplements. My new healthy lifestyle has made such a change in me that my family is amazed. All my prescription drugs are reduced by half and can eventually be eliminated. If my symptoms start to return, I refer back to the program to fine-tune my routine and make use of natural remedies you recommend. Thanks.

PART THREE

THE CUSTOMIZED PLANS

14

FOR THOSE OVER AGE FIFTY

BY AGE FIFTY, we are solidly in middle age, no longer young, at significant risk for cardiovascular disease and other illnesses. Women experience menopause and may face an "empty-nest syndrome," with children grown and gone. We may watch parents die or suffer from progressive, chronic ailments that conventional medicine can do little to change, and we may begin to think seriously about our own eventual decline. Yet these years should be the prime of life. Middle-aged bodies may be less flexible, less resilient, and more likely to annoy us, but if we dedicate ourselves to protecting and enhancing our natural healing potentials, our bodies can also be radiantly healthy.

If you have not followed the steps of the Eight-Week Program earlier in life, now is the time to begin.

Projects

• This would be a good occasion to get a medical checkup if you have not had one recently. It should include a full history and physical examination, with particular attention to any new complaints or symptoms. Blood work should include a complete blood count, general blood chemistries (a "SMAC-20"), and a serum-lipid profile that reveals not only total cholesterol but its breakdown into HDL, LDL, and other fractions, as well as serum triglycerides. The examination should also include urinalysis and a stool sample to detect any abnormal bleeding, and an electrocardiogram. If there is any reason to suspect heart disease, a cardiac-stress (treadmill) test should be done. Men should have two prostate checks: a digital rectal examination, and a blood test for PSA, the antigen whose elevation can indicate early prostate cancer. Women should have a mammogram in addition to the regular gynecological examination and Pap smear. If they have a family history of osteoporosis or fit the physical profile of susceptibility to that disease, bone-density testing is also advisable. Many medical experts recommend sigmoidoscopy for both men and women by age fifty as a screen for early colon cancer, which is reliably curable (by surgery) only if it is discovered while still localized.

• It is also not a bad idea to go for fitness testing, including assessment of body composition, strength, flexibility, and aerobic capacity. This can be done at some medical facilities, health clubs, or spas. Keep all of this information in an accessible file in case you need to consult a doctor for any future problems.

• Please work at all of the other projects in the basic Eight-Week Program. This is a good time in life to begin taking one of the tonics described in Week Six. All of these natural products have the potential to strengthen your healing system and protect it from some of the decreasing efficiency that comes with aging.

Diet

I observe that, as people in our culture grow older, they naturally tend to select lighter, healthier food, often eating less red meat in favor of more fish and chicken, for example. Whether this results from a change in digestion or greater awareness of the relationship between diet and health I do not know. In any case, if you do not now follow the dietary guidelines of the program, please start doing so. I can promise you that you will notice significant changes in how you feel, with more energy and greater vitality.

• Pay particular attention to the amount of fat you eat. In middle age, metabolism slows, and weight not only goes on faster, it comes off much less easily. I usually recommend that no more than 25 percent of calories come from fat, and of course you want to keep your saturated-fat intake as low as possible. This is a good time in life to leave behind the dietary excesses of youth.

Supplements

The antioxidant formula is of great importance in middle age, a kind of insurance against some of the hazards of old age.

• If you are taking a multivitamin or some other supplement, read the label carefully to determine how much of the four components of the formula it is giving you, and make up for any deficiencies by taking extra amounts. There is no problem in taking a multivitamin in addition to the formula.
• Be sure to get 800 IU of natural vitamin E daily.

Exercise

I hope you have not waited until now to start exercising, but if that is the case, the walking that is part of the program is the best possible activity for you, much better than running or playing competitive sports. Your body is more susceptible to injury after age fifty, so it is important to pick a form of exercise that carries a low risk of injury, one that you can stick with through the years. If you engage in more vigorous aerobic activity, this may be a good time to shift some of your energy into brisk daily walks.

• If you are not in the habit of stretching, go gently and easily with this recommendation at first. You may find it harder to stretch in the morning, easier in the afternoon or evening. Try it before you go to bed. Increasing your flexibility is one of the best ways to condition your musculoskeletal system and reduce the chance of serious injury if you suffer a fall or are in an accident.

Mental/Spiritual

• As you watch parents and others deal with serious illness, it is easy to become pessimistic about health and healing. Resist that trend by continuing to focus on healing experiences in yourself, family, and friends.
• It is a perfectly realistic goal to experience old age with all of your faculties intact and your body still giving you good service. You can

increase that probability by following all of the steps of the Eight-Week Program, especially those aimed at enhancing your mental and spiritual health.

• Middle age is often a time of great engagement with the world, the phase of life when professional and vocational accomplishment is greatest, social responsibilities are most pressing, and leisure time is scarce. Therefore, it is also the time when you need to be skillful at relaxing, neutralizing stress, and renewing yourself. The mental/spiritual exercises of the Eight-Week Program can be very helpful to you in your prime, making you more effective in the world, as well as happier and healthier.

• Set a good example for the people you come in contact with. People who ignore the principles of healthy living often begin to pay for their folly in middle age. Your embodiment of health in the prime of your life will inspire others to take more responsibility for their own well-being.

15

FOR THOSE OVER AGE SEVENTY

MOST PEOPLE ASSOCIATE OLD AGE with sickness and infirmity, but all of us have met individuals who retain vigor, vitality, and beauty into their eighties and nineties. Clearly, genetic inheritance plays a role in shaping how we age. I believe that lifestyle is also important, because some of the very healthy old people I know have lived longer and aged better than their parents, who did not have access to the kind of information in the Eight-Week Program and went along with cultural trends of the past. At whatever age you begin to follow these recommendations, the healthier lifestyle you create will serve you well as you advance in years.

What changes in us as we age? Some aspects of myself seem not much different now from when I was in my twenties. I assume that my spiritual self is unaffected by passing time; indeed, an essential quality of spirit is independence of space and time even when it is invested in the physical world. What has changed greatly is my physical body. My metabolism, sleep patterns, reactions to stimuli, and, of course, my external appearance are all quite different from what they were in my youth. Certainly, those external changes are mirrored in changes throughout the internal structure of my body, and if I were simply to focus on the general graying, wrinkling, and stiffening that aging brings to the body, I could let myself become depressed and anxious.

One of the great challenges of life is to come to terms with physical decline and death. One way to work at that is to practice observing the changes that time brings dispassionately, without reacting to them with denial or aversion. From this perspective, the aging of the physical body is just change—interesting, neutral change that may dictate adjustment of one's activities but is of no particular import on the mental/spiritual level. A traditional Buddhist practice is meditation in the presence of corpses or in graveyards, not out of any morbid fascination with death, but as a technique to decondition reflexive aversion to the inevitable decay of physical form. Here is a contemporary Buddhist, the Vietnamese meditation teacher Thich Nhat Hanh, reflecting on this practice:

> When I was only 19 years old, I was assigned by an older monk to meditate on the image of a corpse in the cemetery. But I found it very hard to take and resisted the meditation. Now I no longer feel that way. Then I thought that such a meditation should be reserved for older monks. But since then, I have seen many young soldiers lying motionless beside one another, some only 13, 14, and 15 years old. They had no preparation or readiness for death. Now I see that if one doesn't know how to die, one can hardly know how to live— because death is a part of life.

As you enter the ultimate decades of your life, it is necessary to health and happiness to be at peace with the aging of your body. I have added some appropriate recommendations to the mental/spiritual section of the program, which I hope will help you in this regard.

I would also ask you to look at your relationship with professional medicine and doctors. In this period of life, most people see doctors more frequently, and many require treatment for chronic conditions, but it is all too easy to become overly dependent on medical intervention, particularly on drugs. When I look in the medicine cabinets of elderly friends and relatives, the usual sight that greets me is a very large array of bottles of prescribed medication. Many of these people are on five or more drugs at once, with high risk of adverse reactions and interactions.

Projects

• Make a point of seeking out persons who are aging well. Use them as role models and talk to them about ways they have found to adjust to the changes in their bodies and keep themselves optimally healthy.

• Go through your medicine cabinet and look at all the drugs you keep there. Are they all necessary? Might there be alternative, more natural ways of managing some of the conditions for which they were prescribed? Use the resource guide listed in the appendix to help you with this project.

Diet

The digestive systems of many older people work more slowly and are less tolerant of abuse than those of younger people. The general dietary advice of the program applies to you, but it is especially important that you maintain a good intake of fiber by eating whole-grain products and an abundance of fruits and vegetables. Many older people find that they no longer care for meals heavy with animal protein and rich sauces. Unfortunately, many older people also find themselves in institutions where the meals served to them do not reflect the orientation of this program. If that is the case (similar, by the way, to the problem young people face in school cafeterias), you must learn to make wise choices from what is offered.

Remember that, to maintain regular eliminations, you must drink enough water and get adequate exercise as well as pay attention to intake of fiber.

• If constipation is a problem, use an herbal bowel-regulator from India called *triphala,* a mainstay of Ayurvedic medicine that is now available in health-food stores here. Triphala is a mixture of three fruits that tones the musculature of the GI system without acting as an irritant laxative. It is intended for regular use, not for symptomatic treatment, and has greater benefit the longer you use it.

Supplements

• Use one (or more) of the tonics described in Week Six. People in your phase of life can most realize the benefits of these gifts of nature, which can tone your healing system, give you more energy, and increase your resistance to infection and stress.
• If you suffer from any deficiency of circulation, consider using ginkgo, the extract of the leaves of a tree (*Ginkgo biloba*) that is widely used in Germany to increase blood flow throughout the body.

Ginkgo is nontoxic and not an anticoagulant; it may work by increasing the elasticity of the membranes of red blood cells, making it easier for them to squeeze through small arteries and capillaries. Many people report both physical and mental improvement after using this herbal remedy for at least two months. You will find standardized extracts in tablet form in health-food stores. The dose is 40 milligrams three times a day with meals.

• Add a calcium supplement to your vitamin-and-mineral regimen if you do not already take one. Women begin to lose bone density in middle age; men lose it later in life, but by their late seventies and early eighties are equally at risk for osteoporosis. Supplemental calcium definitely helps. Take 1,000 to 1,500 milligrams of calcium citrate, the form most easily absorbed, at bedtime, preferably with a tablespoon of nonfat or low-fat cottage cheese or the same amount of tofu or another form of soy protein to enhance absorption. Be aware that calcium is constipating. To avoid that effect, take it with magnesium, which is laxing and balances calcium's effects in other ways: 500 to 1,000 milligrams of magnesium gluconate, chelate, or citrate. Pay attention to bowel function to find the ratio of the two minerals that is right for you.

Exercise

• Don't neglect the walking. It is the perfect activity for older bodies.
• Keep up your stretching. The more you maintain flexibility, the lower your chance of injury.
• If you suffer from arthritis or have any problems with joints or muscles, try to spend some time in comfortably warm water. Swimming, water aerobics for seniors, or just paddling around in your own style are all good for your musculoskeletal system.

Mental/Spiritual

• I would like you to consider this "exercise in mindfulness" from Thich Nhat Hanh.

Lie on a bed, or on a mat or on the grass in a position in which you are comfortable. Don't use a pillow. Begin to take hold of your breath. Imagine all that is left of your body is a white skeleton lying on the face of the earth. Maintain [a] half smile and continue to follow your breath. Imagine that all your flesh has decomposed and is gone, that your skeleton is now lying in the earth 80 years after burial. See clearly the bones of your head, back, your ribs, your hip bones, leg and arm bones, finger bones. Maintain the half smile, breathe very lightly, your heart and mind serene. See that your skeleton is not you. Be at one with life. Live eternally in the trees and grass, in other people, in the birds and other beasts, in the sky, in the ocean waves. Your skeleton is only one part of you. You are present everywhere and in every moment. You are not only a bodily form, or even feelings, thoughts, actions, and knowledge.

Thich Nhat Hanh recommends doing this exercise for twenty to thirty minutes at a time. Try it first for just a few minutes to see if you can ease into such unfamiliar mental territory.
• When you practice Breath Observation, try to identify with your breath as your unchanging essence, the connection with the aspect of your being that does not age and does not die.
• Take full satisfaction in having reached the maturity of human experience and wisdom and retained interest in and dedication to living in optimum health.

16

FOR THOSE UNDER AGE TWENTY

I WANT TO BEGIN by commending you on taking interest in preventive health maintenance at a young age. Chances are that your body is serving you very well. You have probably had some infectious illnesses in childhood, the usual colds, and perhaps some allergies, but the major threat to your health has probably been physical trauma, accidents you have suffered that I hope you have recovered from quickly and completely. Your healing potential is high, and if you begin to protect it now, it will serve you well for the rest of your life.

Projects

• Follow the program exactly as it is presented. The only suggestion that may not be important for you is the one concerning tonics. If you are generally healthy, your healing system is already well toned and resilient and does not need an herbal boost. In general, older people need these aids more, and there may be a danger of squandering their power if you use them too early in life in the absence of need. A Chinese pharmacologist, who was quite devoted to the subject, once told me, "Do not waste ginseng in your youth; save it for old age, and then see what it can do for you."
• Take seriously all of the recommendations about protection from toxins. If you follow them, you will have a great advantage over people who do not begin to worry about this issue until they are in middle age or beyond. Toxic damage to the body's healing system is the result of multiple low-level exposures over time from various sources.

Start taking protective measures now, and by the time you are older, your cumulative exposure will be much less than that of many of your contemporaries.

Diet

• Try to adhere to the dietary recommendations of the program. The earlier in life you can begin to follow them the better, because the damage done to the body by unhealthy food choices, like that done by toxins, results from long-term, cumulative exposure. As an example, consider the risk of atherosclerosis and its relationship to high serum cholesterol, resulting, in most cases, from eating too much saturated fat. Babies need more fat than the rest of us and can process the saturated fat of breast milk, but starting at age three the effects of high intake of saturated fat in milk and meat products become evident, appearing at first as yellowish streaks in the intimal lining of coronary arteries. By late adolescence, many boys in our society have significant coronary atherosclerosis, although it will be years before arterial flow decreases to the point where symptoms appear. (Keep in mind that the first symptom of this disease of lifestyle may be a fatal heart attack.) This fact was sadly apparent in the autopsy findings on young American soldiers killed in recent wars.

I will acknowledge that you face greater obstacles than your elders in implementing the dietary changes of the program. You may not always be in control of your food, especially if you live at home, attend school away from home, or live on your own with little experience of food preparation and little inclination to cook for yourself. If you live at home, you might try to get your parents on the Eight-Week Program, or at least to take an interest in its dietary recommendations. Maybe you can set a healthy example for the rest of your family that they will eventually follow.

Institutional kitchens serve up a great deal of unhealthy as well as unappetizing food, especially too many animal products, poorly cooked vegetables, and too much of the wrong kinds of fats. Fast-food establishments are easy and cheap, and cater to the tastes of young people; the food they serve is very high in the wrong kinds of fats.

If you eat in institutional dining halls, you will have to learn to choose wisely from what is offered. Avoid deep-fried foods, for example, cut back on meats, select whole-wheat bread over white, try to eat the vegetables, and consider supplementing your diet with garlic, ginger, and occasional soy burgers.

Another problem you might run into is feeling antisocial or different as a result of your interest in healthy eating. Sharing meals and snack foods with friends is a major way of socializing while you are growing up, and it may be hard to pass up the foods that others want to eat. Please be flexible. Your body can handle a certain amount of junk food. Your real aim is to develop—gradually if necessary—healthy habits of eating that will serve you over your lifetime. I promise you that it is possible to get as much pleasure—or even more pleasure—from foods that contribute to your health as from the foods that most people learn to crave in our society.

Supplements

• Make the antioxidant formula a part of your daily routine. The earlier in life you begin taking antioxidant vitamins and minerals, the longer they will work for you as you age. You only need 400 IU of natural vitamin E; the rest of the formula stays the same.

Exercise

• The earlier in life you develop solid, sensible habits of exercise, the easier it will be for you to maintain them, even though the circumstances of your life change greatly. Think about your level of physical activity. Most of us assume that young people are physically active, but all of the surveys I have seen suggest that American children are more sedentary than ever, with television and computers likely contributing causes. Since your body probably does not bother you much at this age, it may not make its need for exercise directly known to you. Older people may have an advantage here, because they can often feel immediate benefits from exercising as well as the effects of skipping it.

• Many young people I meet cannot see the wisdom of walking, considering it too mild to count as exercise. They would rather play competitive sports, run, or pump weights. If you like those activities, do them. Just consider what I have said about walking as the best form of exercise and try to do more rather than less of it whenever you can. And practice stretching. You are much more flexible now than you will be in thirty years; not only is stretching easier for you than for me, but if you develop it as a habit at this point in your life, you will retain much more flexibility in later life than many of your contemporaries.

Mental/Spiritual

• You are in a good position to observe your body's healing system at work whenever you sustain an injury or have an infection. In most cases, healing in young people is swift and sure. Learn to see it for what it is and to appreciate it. Building confidence about your healing ability at a young age will also serve you well.

I have no other modifications to suggest in the mental/spiritual components of the basic program. They are as important for young people as for anyone else. It is never too early to begin learning how to value the needs and interests of others.

Finally, let me say again that your decision to follow the Eight-Week Program is commendable. If more people in your age group would do so, we would be a healthier society with far smaller expenditures for doctors, medicines, and hospital stays.

17

FOR MEN

MEN IN OUR CULTURE have shorter lifespans than women, often succumb in their forties and fifties to heart attacks, are more prone to violence, accidental injury, and death, and tend to be more constricted emotionally than their female counterparts. They are also less likely to ask for help, whether for directions or for interpretations of symptoms; as a result they often ignore or deny medical problems, and use health professionals only as last resorts. Because of these and other risks, I believe that men need to pay special attention to particular aspects of the Eight-Week Program. Here are the modifications I suggest.

Projects

• Read the above paragraph again. Can you identify with any of the problem behavioral patterns common to your gender? If so, make a list of them and think about ways you can change them within the context of the program. They are obstacles to your progress toward optimum health.

• Think about the sources of stress in your life that have to do with being a man. You may have to be the main provider for a family, to spend many hours in a competitive workplace, and feel compelled to achieve or live up to impossible standards. Do you have close male friends you can share your anxieties and frustrations with? If not, make a resolution to try to develop such friendships.

Diet

In my experience as a physician, I have found men more likely than women to be stuck in meat-and-potatoes patterns of eating, to be especially enamored of oversized portions of beef, and to reject vegetables, except for salads doused in high-fat dressings. Some men regard soy foods and other vegetarian main dishes as unmanly, an attitude that is fine if you consider it manly to exit the world prematurely.

• Make a special effort to adhere to the dietary recommendations in this program, especially with regard to reducing consumption of animal foods and increasing consumption of fresh fruits and vegetables.
• Know the sources of saturated fat in your diet and keep them to a minimum. Cheese accounts for a great deal of the saturated fat in the Western diet, and the fatty-acid spectrum of beef fat is particularly unhealthy for the heart and arteries.
• Eat tomatoes and tomato products regularly; the lycopene in them is protective against prostate cancer, a major health risk for men as they age.

Supplements

• If you take a multivitamin-and-mineral supplement, be sure that it does not contain iron. Men have no way to eliminate iron except through blood loss, and high levels of it in the body may promote cardiovascular disease and cancer.
• Some of the tonics described in Week Six are particularly esteemed by men in Asia. That is true of Asian ginseng and ashwagandha, for example, both of which have a reputation as enhancers of male sexual vigor in addition to their general effects on resistance, skin and muscle tone, and healing. Consider using them if you experience a decline in sexuality.
• Most men over fifty develop benign enlargement of the prostate, the walnut-sized gland that surrounds the urethra at the neck of the bladder. This enlargement is influenced by hormonal metabolism and is not a precursor of malignant change; however, it can decrease the force of the urinary stream and lead to increased urinary frequency, nighttime urination, and other symptoms. A safe and effective herbal

remedy for this condition is saw palmetto, prepared from the fruit of a small palm tree (*Serenoa repens*) native to the Atlantic coast of North America from South Carolina to Florida. It is less toxic than the pharmaceutical drugs most doctors prescribe for prostatic enlargement and widely available in health-food stores, often combined with another useful herb, *Pygeum africanum,* and various vitamins and minerals. Use a standardized extract of saw palmetto and take about 160 milligrams twice a day; you can use this product safely over a long period of time.

• Resist the temptation to take hormonal "fountains of youth" like growth hormone, DHEA (a male sex hormone), and melatonin, some of which are sold alongside vitamins and minerals in health-food stores. Hormones are powerful bioregulators with very general effects on the body; in most cases, the consequences of long-term supplementation with these substances are not known.

Exercise

• Pay attention to your body, listen to its complaints, and stop any activities that bother it. It is a shame to see young men out of action with damaged knees, shoulders, and backs as a result of playing football and other intense, competitive sports. There is a time and place for such activities, but I know many men who are unwilling to give them up as they age, even as their bodies become less forgiving of physical abuse. "Running through the pain" has left many men unable to run at all, and some unable to do any exercise.

• Walking as a form of exercise is never to be dismissed lightly. I predict that fitness research will demonstrate it to be superior even to running as a general conditioner.

• Avoid the common male pattern in our society of being active and athletic in youth, only to be sedentary in middle age. It is much better to stick with a regular, moderate, sensible form of exercise that will hold up throughout your life.

Mental/Spiritual

It has become a cliché that men have trouble expressing their feelings, but in fact many of them learn to think that admitting to vulnerability or emotional pain is a sign of weakness and therefore not masculine.

Of course, some men express some emotions all too readily: rage when frustrated, for example, which not only accounts for their dispropor- tionate representation as perpetrators of violence but also seems to be a risk factor for heart attack.

• If you have difficulty controlling anger, put special effort into work- ing with the Relaxing Breath that I taught you. Also try to extend your periods of Breath Observation into a formal meditation prac- tice—say, for twenty to thirty minutes a day. You may find that yoga will help you to eliminate violent reactions as well; it also more than satisfies your body's need for healthy stretching.

• If you have difficulty knowing or expressing your feelings, consider some individual or group psychotherapy, or try attending a men's group that suits your tastes. Men who learn to be more comfortable with and expressive of emotions are healthier as well as happier.

• Work on developing meaningful connections: with your fellow men, with your family, friends, neighbors, pets, plants, and the earth. Because men are more likely than women to see themselves as self- contained and pride themselves on being independent, they are also more likely than women to suffer from the Disconnection Syndrome I wrote about in Week Seven. Unmarried men are more likely to have problems with substance abuse than their married counterparts and are more likely to get sick and die young. In many parts of the world, violence is mostly committed by lone males. Connect!

18

FOR WOMEN

THE FEMALE REPRODUCTIVE SYSTEM is much more complicated than the male and creates particular health risks for women. For example, female reproductive-system cancers are common and life-threatening; they are also increasing in frequency throughout the world, probably as a result of increased exposure to pollutants that act like estrogens, as I explained in Week Two. It is vitally important that you do everything in your power to reduce your risks of these terrible diseases. Women are also much more likely than men to develop autoimmunity (as in rheumatoid arthritis and lupus), Alzheimer's disease, and osteoporosis. It is in your interest to learn about your body and the breakdowns to which you are predisposed by heredity. You can then take preventive action.

Although women are less likely than men to be cut off from their feelings or unable to express them, they are more likely to suffer from depression and to receive pharmaceutical treatment for emotional disorders. Since the beginning of the modern psychopharmaceutical industry in the middle of this century, women have been far and away the main target population for all the tranquilizers, stimulants, and antidepressants, many of them addictive and unhealthy in long-term usage. As the main caretakers in society, women often have to meet impossible demands. Those who try to work in male-dominated businesses and professions get paid less for equivalent work and may have to develop a competitive edge that subjects them to damaging stress. In many societies women still must contend with a predominant attitude that their only appropriate roles outside the home are as schoolteachers and nurses.

Women generally ask for help with much less difficulty than men and so find it easier to consult with health professionals about symptoms, but, given the nature of allopathic medicine today, they are also more likely to hear their complaints dismissed as "hysterical," or to wind up being dependent on practitioners, both conventional and alternative. In midlife, women face a major biological change—menopause—that men do not have to deal with. It raises many emotional and medical concerns, such as fears of losing youthful attractiveness and sexual appeal and worries about the safety of the hormone-replacement therapy that is urged upon them by most doctors.

Because for many women attracting men is a top priority, concerns about appearance and sexual attractiveness are major motivators. In societies that extol anorexic leanness as the ideal of feminine beauty, women can easily drive themselves to distraction with diets and exercise regimens that in no way promote health; they are also easy marks for the advertising efforts of manufacturers of cosmetic and beauty products. I know the pressures you face, because I have seen too many women's-magazine covers that advertise the latest crash diets right next to pictures of tempting chocolate cakes you are encouraged to make from recipes inside. A major reason for the extent of tobacco addiction among women today is that girls learn to use cigarettes for comfort in place of sweets and other fattening foods; most of them live in fear of getting fat if they quit. And, as I'm sure you know, women are many times more likely to develop eating disorders than men. Learning to like your body and treat it well may be harder for you than it is for most men, but it is essential if you are to avoid the pitfall of pursuing an impossible body image.

Compared with men, women are more likely to be knowledgeable about alternatives to standard medicine, more willing to experiment with herbal remedies, more likely to engage in counseling and psychotherapy, more informed about nutrition, more enthusiastic about eating fruits, vegetables, and foods other than meat and potatoes. Women's magazines have been major sources of information about natural therapies, and throughout the world it is women who are taking the lead in the consumers' movement that is beginning to change medical institutions and practice. This is also a big responsibility: you may have to inspire, cajole, or push your mate in the direction of healthier living.

Here are some additions and modifications of the Eight-Week Program just for you:

Projects

• Read over the above paragraphs again and see if you identify with any of the common problems and challenges of women today. If so, think about how you are coping with them and what else you can do to alleviate them.
• Compile a brief medical history of your female blood relatives: sisters, mother, mother's sisters, maternal grandmother. Are there any diseases that stand out in this group? If so, read up on them and the lifestyle factors that might influence them.
• Look up the resources on women's health listed in the appendix of this book. Make a point of using some of them to expand your knowledge of your body.
• Be diligent about protecting yourself from toxins in water, food, and your environment, as the program suggests. Many pollutants have the potential to increase your risk of breast cancer and other disorders of your reproductive system.
• Go through your cosmetic products (including shampoos) and identify those containing artificial coloring. When you use them up, try to find alternatives that are uncolored or contain only natural coloring agents.

Diet

• Be sure to get adequate intake of food sources of omega-3 fatty acids, as described in Week One. Their natural anti-inflammatory effect will protect you from many of the conditions women are more prone to develop.
• If you eat much meat, poultry, and dairy products, make an effort to get organic products, certified to be free of hormones (which are estrogenic and add to the hormonal load on cells in your breasts, ovaries, and uterus).

• Be sure to make soybean products a regular part of your diet as another defense against estrogenic pressures.

• Pay attention to the latest research findings on the health risks of alcohol. There is growing realization that, because alcohol affects the body's production and use of estrogen, even moderate intake may significantly raise the risk of breast cancer in susceptible women.

• Although your hormones protect you from coronary heart disease until menopause, it is never too early to begin following a heart-healthy diet that is low in saturated fat and high in fruits and vegetables.

• Get regular gynecological checkups, including periodic Pap smears to detect early cervical cancer. Learn to examine your breasts yourself each month, and get a baseline mammogram by age fifty. If you are at risk for osteoporosis because of your body type (light-boned, fair skin) or family history, have your bone density measured before you go through menopause, and if it is below normal, consult with your physician about ways of slowing or reversing bone loss.

• Hormone-replacement therapy significantly reduces risk of coronary heart disease in women, slows bone loss, protects against Alzheimer's disease, and prevents menopausal symptoms. Also, however, it can increase risks of female reproductive cancers. To make an informed decision about it, you must weigh the benefits against the risks, based on your past medical and family history, the availability of alternatives, and your willingness to make lifestyle changes. See the appendix for more information on this subject.

• Be sure to avoid the use of artificial sweeteners and products containing them.

Supplements

• Add a calcium supplement to the basic formula: 1,000 to 1,500 milligrams of calcium citrate, the form most easily absorbed, at bedtime, preferably with a tablespoon of nonfat or low-fat cottage cheese or the same amount of tofu or other form of soy protein to enhance absorption further. Also take it with 500 to 1,000 milligrams of magnesium (gluconate, chelate, or citrate), because the two minerals balance each other.

• There are a number of good tonic herbs for women, such as dong quai, which I described in Week Six. Traditional Chinese medicine also has good herbal formulas that harmonize and tone the female reproductive organs.

Exercise

• If men often form unhealthy exercise habits because they become obsessed with physical fitness, women often do the same for weight control. Try to avoid damaging your body by working it too hard, and don't slight walking as the best exercise.

Mental/Spiritual

• If you are prone to emotional instability, work diligently with the breathing exercises of the Eight-Week Program. Over time they will help even out your moods.
• Do not hesitate to seek help from counselors and therapists if you experience emotional problems.
• Experiment with visualization as a healing technique, as described in Week Two. Women are often very talented in this area, and if you develop this skill, it will help you avoid becoming dependent on medical interventions and practitioners.
• Also explore the various forms of touch healing, such as therapeutic touch, which is mostly practiced by nurses, or reiki, jin shin jyutsu, and other forms of energy transfer through the hands. Women often learn these techniques more readily than men, and all of them are valuable. Check the appendix for sources of information and training.

19

FOR PREGNANT WOMEN (AND THOSE CONSIDERING PREGNANCY)

PREGNANCY OFFERS THE CHANCE to give a new human being the best possible start to a healthy life. It also creates special needs for a woman's body that dictate modification of some of the steps of the Eight-Week Program.

Projects

• Find out about techniques of "conscious conception and birth" to increase the likelihood of problem-free pregnancy and birth as well as the production of an optimally healthy baby in all senses of the word. A good source of information is *The Child of Your Dreams* by Laura Archera Huxley and Piero Ferrucci, now, unfortunately, out of print. Among other methods, the authors recommend that you and your mate talk regularly to the developing baby and play harmonious music to it through the abdominal wall.

• Consider the use of professional midwives to assist you in both pregnancy and delivery. I am a strong proponent of home birth, natural childbirth, and midwife-assisted delivery. I also encourage the use of hospital birthing centers that welcome midwives and allow natural childbirth in medical settings.

• Maintain the best possible general health, using the Eight-Week Program as a general guide.

• Discontinue use of all drugs, prescribed and over-the-counter, medical or recreational, legal or illegal (unless your physician deems them necessary). The developing fetus is very vulnerable to pharmacological influences, especially during the first three months, when organs are being formed. Even moderate amounts of alcohol and coffee can affect development, for example. For the same reason, avoid herbal remedies as much as possible.

• Ask your doctor about the sweat bathing recommended in Week Five. I advise pregnant women against soaking in hot tubs, but I agree with Finnish physicians that moderate use of sauna is not a problem in pregnancy. If you like to sweat bathe, talk the issue over with your doctor or midwife.

Diet

• Protein needs are somewhat increased in pregnancy, but not as much as you would think. Do not feel compelled to drink milk or eat more meat unless you have clear cravings for such foods. In general, listen to your body; it will tell you what it needs.

• Avoid or reduce intake of strongly flavored foods and pungent spices (like black pepper and mustard, for example). An interesting theory sees morning sickness as a protective reaction to minimize exposure of the embryo to potentially toxic agents that might cause developmental abnormalities. Pay attention to what makes you queasy, and listen also to what your body tells you it does not want.

• If you do experience morning sickness, the safest remedy is application of a wrist band that stimulates an acupuncture point controlling nausea. (See the appendix for sources.) You can also try taking ginger in the form of tea or capsules; it works and is safer than any drug your doctor can prescribe.

• Be diligent about following the guidelines of the program for minimizing exposure to toxins from water and food.

• In the last month of pregnancy and first month of neonatal life, omega-3 fatty acids are rapidly incorporated into the brain of the baby. Be sure to include extra amounts of salmon, sardines, or flax into your diet during this period. (The omega-3s you eat will pass into your breast milk.)

Supplements

• Your doctor should be able to recommend a good prenatal vitamin-and-mineral supplement containing extra iron and calcium.

• Folic acid, a B vitamin, is now known to prevent neural tube defects like spina bifida, a serious abnormality of early fetal development. Unfortunately, by the time most women learn they are pregnant, the critical period has already passed. A major source of folic acid is the cooked greens recommended in the program (another is orange juice). If you are contemplating pregnancy or think there is any possibility that you could get pregnant, for insurance take a daily B-complex vitamin supplement providing 400 micrograms of folic acid.

• Your baby's teeth will be forming during the latter half of pregnancy. If you provide them with a low dose of fluoride during this period, the benefits on permanent dental health will be great. If you follow the recommendation of the Eight-Week Program to purify your drinking water (or use bottled water), you will not be getting fluoride even though your water supply contains it. Your doctor can prescribe a liquid or tablet form of fluoride for use as a daily supplement and can tell you the correct dose (1 milligram a day is usual). Continue the supplement while you are nursing. I am very aware of the controversy surrounding fluoride and fluoridation of public water supplies; as with most medical treatments, there are both risks and benefits here, which I believe to be dose-related. In appropriate doses the benefits of fluoride far outweigh the risks. My wife followed this recommendation in all but one of her pregnancies, and the difference is obvious in the child who did not get the supplement.

• Check the amounts of vitamins C and E, beta-carotene, and selenium provided in your prenatal multivitamin-and-mineral supplement. Adjust the antioxidant formula so that you do not ingest more than the recommended daily doses. Those doses are fine to continue through your pregnancy.

• Do not use any of the herbal tonics described in Week Six.

Exercise

• Your birth experience will be easier if you are in good physical condition and can use your voluntary muscles to assist uterine contractions during delivery. Some women runners and athletes have difficulty with this, because the tone of their voluntary muscles is too high, and they cannot relax enough to work in synchrony with the uterus. This is another reason to develop moderate, sensible habits of exercise.

• You can continue the walking right up to your due date. It will help you maintain normal weight, digestion, and muscle tone throughout pregnancy.

• Stretching is also a good way to keep your muscles toned during pregnancy, even though you will have to modify your routine as your body contour changes.

• If back pain is a problem in the later months, try a few sessions of chiropractic or osteopathic manipulative therapy.

Mental/Spiritual

• The breath work of the program is excellent preparation for childbirth. All systems of natural childbirth stress breath control as the most important way to adjust to the pain of uterine contractions and keep body and mind in the right state during labor and delivery. Especially practice the relaxing breath.

• Exposing yourself to flowers, beauty, music, and art in order to uplift your spirits while you are pregnant affects the consciousness of your baby as well.

• The second stage of labor, in which the baby begins to traverse the birth canal, is marked by a profoundly altered state of consciousness, one that many women report to be a peak experience. This is one of the main reasons for preparing to deliver without the use of drugs that dull perception. You have an opportunity here for catching a glimpse of the threshold between the material and the spiritual world.

• Visualization therapy and hypnotherapy can be powerful tools to assist you during pregnancy and birth. If you have problems during pregnancy or feel you need help preparing for childbirth, find a therapist you feel comfortable working with who is skilled in these methods. They are harmless and can be remarkably effective, even in one or two sessions. In *Spontaneous Healing* I told the story of my wife, Sabine, who three weeks before her due date did a session of hypnotherapy to ask the baby to come on time and to turn from its posterior presentation. The baby did so within twenty minutes of the request and was born right on schedule. You will find information on these therapies in the appendix.

20

FOR PARENTS OF YOUNG CHILDREN

PARENTING IS AN ULTIMATE CHALLENGE and ultimate reward. I ask you to consider two aspects of it: how the presence of young children in your home may affect your ability to follow the steps of the Eight-Week Program, and how you can take advantage of opportunities to encourage your children to begin developing healthy habits earlier rather than later in life.

An infant requires frequent attention and often dramatically interferes with its parents' sleep. The arrival of a baby may well add a whole new dimension of stress and anxiety to life, balanced, of course, by the joy of bonding with a new being. Sometimes, pregnancy and birth can motivate parents to clean up their acts: to stop smoking, for example, and to pay more attention to the principles of good nutrition. At other times, the responsibilities of being parents can leave people feeling that they do not have the time or energy to take care of themselves. The fact is that the healthier you are in body, mind, and spirit, the better parent you will be; making time to care for yourself must remain a high priority even if you live with demanding children.

The earlier in life that people begin to lay the foundations of healthy lifestyles, the greater the benefits. The more years you live in a healthy fashion, the greater the likelihood that you will avoid the common pitfalls of middle age and continue to experience good health into old age. Also, good habits of eating, exercising, and relaxing are easily acquired in childhood, usually with much less effort than adults require. The more we can communicate information about healthy living to the very young, the more our whole society will move toward better health and away from dependence on costly medical interventions. Remember that most of the diseases that cause premature death and disability and absorb most of our health-care dollars are diseases of lifestyle that could be prevented if people at early enough ages would adopt preventive strategies. You have a responsibility to your children to get this information to them in ways that enable them to make use of it.

Projects

• Resolve to follow the steps of the program. If necessary, negotiate with your spouse for time for each of you to exercise, relax, and tend to your spirits. (Playing with your children can be one way for you to exercise, relax, and elevate your spirits all at once.)

• Use the opportunity of living with children to bring the concept of the body's ability to repair itself more into your family's awareness. Healing occurs rapidly in the young, so you can easily observe it. When your children get cuts or scrapes, ask them to watch what happens over the next few days, and use the experience to help them understand that the human body has a healing system, which is their greatest ally in maintaining health.

• Consider the effects of environmental pollution on your own children and make a special effort to protect them by following the recommendations of the program.

• Teach your children about the importance of sun protection and help them understand why, when the sun is at a high angle in the sky, they should stay out of the sun, cover up, or use sunscreens. Significant sunburns in childhood—those that cause the skin to peel—correlate with increased risk of skin cancer in later life, including malignant melanoma.

• Inform yourself about natural alternatives to conventional treatments for such common childhood ailments as middle-ear infections (see the appendix for resources). Too many children in our society are on endless rounds of antibiotics, which not only may not solve the problems for which they are commonly prescribed but also may weaken immunity and resistance.

• On the other hand, I strongly recommend the basic course of childhood immunizations. They are not without risk, but their benefits greatly outweigh those risks. I am familiar with all the anti-immunization arguments and find them weak. Also, I have spent enough time in Third World countries where these diseases still occur to know that their risks are considerably greater than the risks of immunizing against them.

Diet

• You can help your kids resist the commercial pressures to eat fast foods and unhealthy processed foods by explaining to them in language they can understand, and in a nonjudgmental fashion, why the dietary recommendations in this program are better choices. For example, help them see that garishly colored snack foods dyed with synthetic chemicals do not look natural and do not help the body stay healthy. Provide healthy snack foods instead, like baby carrots.
• Remember that arteriosclerosis begins at a very early age. By age three, your children should not be eating excessive fat and should be avoiding the unhealthy fats that I told you about in Week One.
• If you or your spouse has allergies, asthma, eczema, autoimmunity, bronchitis, or sinusitis, or if your child is experiencing frequent colds and ear infections, it is worth experimenting with total elimination of cow's milk in all of its forms. Goat's milk is OK, as is soy milk, but be aware that soy is a common allergen in infants, especially if it is introduced too early. Milk substitutes made from rice and potatoes do not supply protein.
• It is usually not a problem to get kids to eat fruits and fruit juices, but vegetables are another matter. Try to find ways to make vegetables appetizing for them; some recipe suggestions follow.
• Remember that the common unhealthy eating patterns in our society develop in childhood: eating too much fat, sugar, animal protein, and unhealthy processed and fast foods, and consuming insufficient fiber, fruits, and vegetables.

Here are some kid-friendly recipes for you to try:

✂ Stuffed Green Potatoes ✂

3 large baking potatoes
3 stalks broccoli

1/2 teaspoon salt
1 tablespoon olive oil
1–2 tablespoons rice milk or soy milk
2 tablespoons grated Parmesan cheese

1. Scrub the potatoes and make shallow cuts around their middles to make it easier to cut them in half after baking. Bake the potatoes at 400°F. until soft, usually 1 hour, depending on size of potatoes.

2. Meanwhile, cut the ends from the stalks of broccoli and peel some of the outer skin off to make the stems more edible. Steam the broccoli until crunchy-tender and bright green. Drain and chop fine.

3. Cut potatoes in half and scoop out the insides into a bowl. Add the salt, olive oil, and just enough rice or soy milk to allow you to mash potatoes into a smooth paste. Add the Parmesan cheese and the chopped broccoli and mix well.

4. Pile the mixture back into the potato shells, arrange on a baking dish, and heat them to desired temperature.

✎ *Minestrone* ✎

1 tablespoon olive oil
2 large cloves garlic, chopped
1/2 cup chopped onion
6 cups vegetable stock (see pages 89–91) or water
1 small can (6 ounces) tomato paste
1 medium can (16 ounces) crushed tomatoes
3 carrots, peeled and sliced
2 stalks celery, sliced
1/2 pound potatoes, peeled and diced
1 teaspoon dried whole oregano
1 tablespoon dried basil
1/4 cup chopped fresh parsley
1 cup dried pasta (shells, twists, or elbow macaroni)
2 cups cooked beans (kidney, cannellini, garbanzo, or a mixture of these)
grated Parmesan cheese to taste

1. Heat the olive oil in a large pot. Add the garlic and sauté briefly. Add the onion and sauté for 5 minutes.

2. Add vegetable stock (or water), tomato paste, crushed tomatoes, carrots, celery, and potatoes. Bring to a boil, cover, reduce heat, and simmer for 30 minutes.

3. Add the oregano, basil, parsley, pasta, and beans. Cook 30 minutes more. Garnish with grated Parmesan cheese and serve with whole-grain garlic bread.

✌ *Potato Gnocchi* ✌

3 large baking potatoes
1–2 cups unbleached white flour
salt to taste
dash paprika
dash grated nutmeg
2 tablespoons chopped fresh parsley

1. Peel the potatoes, cut in quarters, cover with cold water, bring to a boil, reduce heat, cover, and cook until tender. Drain and mash.

2. To make the gnocchi, for each cup of mashed potato put 1 cup minus 2 tablespoons unbleached white flour in a bowl and mix with salt to taste, dashes of paprika and nutmeg, and the chopped parsley.

3. Add the warm potatoes and knead on a floured surface just until dough is well mixed and not sticky. Let rest for 15 minutes.

4. Roll chunks of dough on floured board into logs about 1 inch thick. Cut into diagonal slices about 3/4 inch thick.

5. Bring a large pot of water to the boil. Add gnocchi. After they rise to the surface, adjust heat and simmer for 10 minutes, uncovered.

6. Drain well and cover with your favorite pasta sauce.

✌ *A Quick Healthy Dessert* ✌

2 ripe bananas
1 package (10.5 ounces) firm, silken tofu, drained

3 tablespoons pure maple syrup
cinnamon to taste

1. In the container of a blender place the bananas, tofu, maple syrup, and cinnamon to taste. Blend until smooth.

2. Serve at once or chill and serve. You can eat this with berries or other fruit or use as a topping for pancakes.

↜ *Banana Bread* ↝

6 or 7 very ripe bananas
1 1/8 cups raw honey
1/3 cup canola oil
2 teaspoons pure vanilla extract
3 cups whole-wheat pastry flour
2 1/2 teaspoons baking soda
1/4 teaspoon salt
1 1/2 cups chopped walnuts or pecans

1. Mash the bananas and mix with the honey, canola oil, and vanilla extract.

2. Sift together the pastry flour (not regular whole-wheat flour), baking soda, and salt. Add the nuts.

3. Blend the two mixtures and divide into 2 lightly oiled loaf pans. Bake at 350°F. for 40 minutes, or until center is set.

↜ *Cocoa-Banana Frozen Dessert* ↝

4 very ripe bananas
4 heaping teaspoons pure unsweetened cocoa powder
1 teaspoon pure vanilla extract
1–2 tablespoons pure maple syrup (optional)

1. Place the bananas in a blender or food processor with the cocoa powder and vanilla extract. If you like, add the maple syrup.

2. Blend until very smooth. Pour into individual cups or small bowls and freeze until just frozen.

✍ *Canyon Ranch Blueberry Soup* ✍

1/3 cup frozen pineapple-juice concentrate, thawed
1 teaspoon fresh lemon juice
2 1/2 cups fresh or unsweetened frozen blueberries
1/2 teaspoon pure vanilla extract

1. In the container of a blender place the pineapple juice, 1/2 cup cold water, the lemon juice, and 1 1/2 cups of the blueberries. Blend until smooth.

2. Pour mixture in a bowl and add the remaining cup of blueberries and the vanilla extract. Mix well and serve cold. (My kids love this.)

Supplements

• You can give children over the age of five half-doses of the antioxidants I recommended for you. They can take them in addition to any multivitamin.

Exercise

• Too many children today are sedentary. Try to restrict the time you let children sit in front of televisions and computers.

• Encourage your children to walk places instead of riding everywhere in cars, to climb stairs instead of taking elevators and escalators, and to find activities they like that get them to use their bodies. Classes in gymnastics, dance, and martial arts are all available for children.

• Young bodies are extremely flexible. See if you can interest your children in yoga or other forms of stretching. The earlier they begin these activities, the longer they will retain flexibility into adult life. Do your stretching with them.

Mental/Spiritual

• Try doing some of the breath work of the program with your kids, especially the Relaxing Breath. Teach it to them so that they can calm themselves down and fall asleep more easily, for example. Breathing together is a pleasurable way to deepen connection with another person.

• Children have great capacity for visual imagination and fantasy. Encourage them to use it in the service of healing—for example, to visualize pain melting away from injuries and warts shrinking into nothingness. You can develop your own self-healing skill by working with your children, and their early acquisition of it will enable them to use it throughout their lives.

• Consider the forms of mental and spiritual "nutrition" that you provide for your children. Do the movies, television programs, and reading you let them take in contribute to or interfere with the way you would like to see them develop? Without being judgmental or heavy-handed, try to expose them to the same healthy influences I have recommended for you.

21

FOR THOSE LIVING IN BIG CITIES

IF, LIKE MOST PEOPLE in the modern world, you live in a big city, you have to contend with particular health hazards. You will find some aspects of the program easier; for example, you can buy a variety of healthy foods, including organic produce, not available in smaller towns; you can easily find health and fitness clubs or yoga and meditation classes, and you have much greater access to cultural resources, like art museums. Although I now live in a rural area, I grew up in a big city (Philadelphia), have lived in several others, and frequently spend time in urban centers. Here are some of the healthful measures I recommend.

Projects

• Toxic exposure in cities may be greater than in the countryside; at least air quality is likely to be worse, and city water is likely to be chlorinated. Consider getting an air filter for your home or apartment and keep protective house plants around. On days when pollution is bad, make a point of spending time in parks, where trees create microenvironments of cleaner air. Definitely use a water-purifying system.

• Noise pollution in cities can be a big problem. Find out about sound-proofing your living space, use a white-noise generator (as described in Week Four) in your bedroom, and try listening to audiotapes when you are out and about.

• Having refuges from the sensory assaults of the city is crucial to good health. Get to know the local parks and quiet places you can visit, such as gardens, chapels, museums, and reading rooms. Make your home or apartment a place of serenity, beauty, and order. At the very least, turn a room or corner of a room into a special quiet place, where you can practice your breathing exercises, meditate, relax, and decompress from the trials of city life.

• The bigger the city you live in, the more practitioners of natural and alternative medicine you will be able to find. Learn the resources you can draw on if you need professional help for a health problem.

Diet

• One difficulty I experience in cities is temptation by restaurants and shops that offer up so much appealing food, not all of it consistent with the philosophy of the program. Search out those that offer kinds of food you want to emphasize in your diet, and make healthy selections from any menus put in front of you. (And don't deny yourself occasional treats.)

Supplements

• Don't neglect the antioxidant formula. It confers some of the best protection you can get against the city's environmental dangers.

• Use one of the immune-boosting tonics, like maitake, reishi, or astragalus. In cities, people live in close proximity and come into contact with each other more frequently than in rural areas. Germs spread easily in dense populations, so give your immune system some help.

Exercise

• Cities often provide wonderful opportunities to walk. Some of the best walks I have ever had have been in San Francisco, where the hills make for great aerobic exercise, and New York, where human diversity never fails to keep me entertained.

• Try climbing stairs in office and apartment buildings instead of always riding elevators and escalators. Even going up a few flights of stairs is a good aerobic workout.

Mental/Spiritual

• Sensory overload is a fact of city life. Use the breathing exercises of the program to help you relax, and consider additional relaxation training if that is not enough. Possibilities include yoga, meditation, biofeedback, or audiotapes that take you through guided relaxation.
• Loneliness in the midst of a big city can be devastating. Read over the advice about connectedness in Week Seven and think about how you can extend meaningful relationships with others into relationships that nourish you spiritually.
• Bring flowers into your living space as often as you can. They are a way of enjoying the beauty of nature even if you feel cut off from it by the inorganic reality of a manmade environment.

22

FOR THOSE WHO TRAVEL FREQUENTLY

TRAVEL CREATES ITS OWN unique stresses and threats to health as well as challenges to maintaining any kind of regular program. It has always been a significant part of my life, but I notice that, as I get older, my tolerance for many of its physical aspects diminishes. I have grown to dislike airports and airplanes, frequent stays in hotels, and all the anxieties of getting from one place to another. If your business requires you to travel frequently, I recommend that you take certain precautions as well as try to adapt the Eight-Week Program to changing circumstances.

Projects

Air travel is unhealthy for a number of reasons. The food served in airports and planes is generally substandard. Flying exposes you to more cosmic radiation than you get on the earth's surface—enough to increase incidence of certain cancers in career pilots and flight attendants. The air quality in planes is dreadful and has declined as airlines have reduced the amount of fresh air pumped into cabins in an effort to cut costs. Long flights are bad for blood circulation (many people get swollen ankles and feet from prolonged sitting) and disrupt biorhythms in proportion to the number of time zones traversed (see the appendix for more information).

• Take your own food on planes whenever possible. Read labels of snacks, cookies, and other packaged foods you are served; most contain hydrogenated fat, and many contain other unhealthy ingredients as well. If you cannot take your own food, eat airline food selectively.

• Never drink plain water on a flight unless it comes from a bottle or a can. You might want to take a large bottle of water with you, since the humidity in planes is low and it is easy to become dehydrated when you fly.

• If you travel internationally, always look for nonsmoking flights, which are becoming more numerous. Smoking sections on international flights should become things of the past, I hope sooner rather than later.

• If the air seems particularly oppressive, complain to flight attendants, and ask that they request the pilot to introduce more fresh air. You can also request a canister of oxygen to make your breathing easier.

• On long flights, get up and walk around as frequently as you can without creating too much disturbance. You can often stand in the galleys of large aircraft. And you can do isometric exercises in your seat to make your muscles feel better.

• If you find that you frequently get coughs or colds after flying, develop the habit of taking an immune-boosting tonic as a preventive measure, starting a day or two before you fly, continuing through the flight and for a day or two afterward. The one that I use is tincture of echinacea, made from the root of the purple coneflower (*Echinacea purpurea* and related species), a popular herbal remedy that you will find in health-food stores. The dose is one dropperful in a little water four times a day. Echinacea is nontoxic and has proven antibiotic, antiviral, and immune-enhancing effects.

• Make sure you are well supplied with good reading or listening for waits in airports. You can also get a surprising amount of walking done in large airports.

• Taking a mask for your eyes and earplugs on long flights might help you get more sleep.

• If you are flying across more than four time zones, you will probably experience some degree of jet lag. The best remedy is melatonin, no more than 1 milligram taken as a sublingual tablet at bedtime at your destination. You may not need more than one dose to reset your biological clock for the new time zone.

• Be sure to pack your antioxidant supplements for your trip in an accessible place, so that you do not omit taking them in transit. Antioxidants are your best protection against radiation exposure while flying at high altitude.

• Always request nonsmoking rooms in hotels and check on the ventilation of your room. If you cannot open a window to admit fresh air, be sure that the air ducts look clean. Often the filters in hotel rooms have not been changed in a long while. If you call the maintenance office, you can usually get a clean air filter installed quickly.

• Try to choose hotels that have fitness facilities in them or can provide you with passes to nearby fitness clubs, where you can use exercise equipment and sweat out accumulated travel toxins in a sauna or steam room. As more business travelers become health-conscious, more hotels are offering these services.

• Buy bottled water for your room or order it from room service. Or travel with one of the portable filters that remove common impurities from tap water.

• In places that you visit frequently, make an effort to cultivate friendships and business relationships with people who share your interest in health.

Diet

Maintaining a good diet while on the road is often difficult, because you are not able to control where, when, and what you eat in the way you can at home. Eating out and trying new and different foods is one of the delights of traveling. It is not the purpose of the program to deny this experience or diminish the pleasures of the table. There is no essential contradiction between healthy food and pleasurable food. Remember that an occasional splurge is not going to hurt you, but if you travel frequently, it is vital to learn how to eat in restaurants without sabotaging your health. Getting restaurant meals that fit the guidelines of the Eight-Week Program is definitely possible. Here are some suggestions:

• Look for restaurants that offer "heart-healthy" entrees that meet the American Heart Association's standards for low content of fat, saturated fat, and cholesterol.

• At fish restaurants, order grilled or broiled fish without added butter or oil and request that sauces be served on the side.

• Choose whole-grain breads if available and try to eat bread without butter. Many restaurants now offer olive oil as an alternative; use it moderately.

• Ask for salad dressings on the side and choose vinaigrettes or simple oil-and-vinegar versions over creamy ones.

• Ask about availability of fresh vegetables and order them steamed or grilled if possible, with any sauces served separately.

• Try to avoid cream-based soups and fried foods.

• For dessert, try to have fruit, fruit sorbets, or other low-fat choices.

• Do not hesitate to ask waiters for help in ordering, or to ask whether the kitchen can prepare special dishes to meet your needs. Calling the restaurant in advance can make this even easier.

• Take healthy, nonperishable snack foods with you on the road. I often travel with crystallized ginger, good high-fiber crackers, and sometimes a bottle of a favorite hot sauce. You can also make a point of visiting natural-food stores to buy items for your hotel room.

Supplements

• Calculate the number of days you will be away and count out the appropriate number of vitamin-and-mineral pills for your trip. Keep these in your carry-on bag, in case you are separated from your checked luggage.

• Stay on one of the tonics recommended in Week Six to help your body adapt to the increased stress of travel.

Exercise

• Do your best to keep up an exercise routine while you are on the road. You can always walk on city streets, in airports, and through parks and shopping malls. Maybe you can take a walk with a business associate instead of sitting in an office.

• If you like to work out in fitness clubs, inquire about their availability and make time in your schedule to use them.

• If you find you are too busy to take a formal exercise break, make an effort to climb some stairs and walk to some of your appointments instead of riding.

Remember that physical exercise not only conditions your body but helps maintain emotional equilibrium through the rigors of travel. It is not a disaster if you abandon your routine for a while, but, again, if you travel frequently, you will want to find ways to satisfy the exercise requirement of the program when you are away from home.

Mental/Spiritual

• Knowing how to relax and neutralize stress is a key to being a happy traveler. Master the relaxing breath so that you can use it to help you through the uncertainties and anxieties of being on the road.
• Take advantage of the cultural and aesthetic resources of new places, and learn what is available in places you visit frequently. I often seek out botanical gardens, for example, or look for interesting lectures, concerts, and theatrical performances in places I visit.
• Order flowers to make a sterile hotel room more friendly.

23

FOR THOSE WHO ARE OVERWEIGHT

THE WESTERN WORLD, led by the United States and Canada, is experiencing an epidemic of obesity of alarming proportions. The two most obvious reasons for it are diet and inactivity, but multiple factors must be at work. More people in our countries are eating more than they have in the past: bigger portions, containing more calories and more fat. They are also eating more fast foods, which are particularly high in fat as well as carbohydrates that predispose to obesity. At the same time, people are less active, walking and exercising less than their grandparents, who did not go everywhere in automobiles or spend hours in front of television sets.

As more and more people join the ranks of the overweight, the disparity between cultural ideals and realities becomes more tense. We admire models and movie stars who are lean, some of them morbidly so, and our medical authorities constantly warn us about the health hazards of carrying excess weight. Obese individuals may experience discrimination if not scorn, adding to their anxieties, which are often motivations to overeat in the first place. Sales of diet products, diet books, and diet plans have always been high; now pharmaceutical drugs that promise easy weight loss are in fashion. One fact is absolutely clear: diets do not work, except temporarily; nor, in my opinion, do the pharmaceutical companies' best products to date; eventually, almost all dieters who use these methods regain all their lost weight, if not more (see the appendix for more information).

I am interested in the genetic basis of obesity and its interaction with environmental factors. It seems to me that many of us have inherited a distant ancestral trait that once stood human populations in good stead: we are quite efficient at taking in calories when they are available and storing them up as fat. Fat is insurance against hard times, protection from periods of sickness and famine. That genetic constitution was surely a survival advantage in past eras, when most people faced unpredictable cycles of feast and famine, but now, with food available all the time, in greater profusion and variety than ever before in history, it works against us.

The biochemical basis of efficient fat storage probably involves insulin, the pancreatic hormone that controls the distribution and utilization of glucose, blood sugar, which is the common energy denominator of metabolism. Adult-onset diabetes is a severe imbalance of this system. It is the common form of the disease, correlated with overweight and inactivity, the result not of decreased production of insulin but of increased resistance to its effects. My guess is that a broad spectrum of insulin resistance exists, with adult-onset diabetes representing one extreme. Many people who cannot control their weight may fall somewhere on this spectrum, and the genes that predispose them to this condition and to obesity probably are the same ones that helped their distant ancestors adjust to marginal food supplies and unpredictable cycles of feast and famine.

You cannot change your genes, but you can change your lifestyle to make them less of a problem. Here are my suggestions:

Projects

• First of all, find out whether you are really overweight and how much of a problem you have. The conventional method—using actuarial tables of ideal weights based on gender and height—is not that accurate. Determination of body composition is much better. Until recently, the standard way of doing this was cumbersome: weighing a person underwater and comparing that value with weight on an ordinary scale. A newer method uses electronic calipers to measure skin thickness at a few points on the body; it is less accurate, because there is greater chance for operator error. An even simpler and very accurate technique using computerized body images is becoming available. It requires only measuring height and weight and taking a few photographs of the body, which are then analyzed by a computer program that rapidly calculates the percentage of body fat. From that figure, you can make a much more accurate decision about whether you should try to lose weight and what your target weight should be. It will probably give you a more realistic goal than the actuarial tables indicate.

• If you are significantly overweight, think about the problems it causes in your life. Is it a health risk? Our doctors, being products of our culture, probably exaggerate the dangers of obesity. If you are active, follow a healthy lifestyle, and have no family history of diseases that correlate with obesity (like adult-onset diabetes and early coronary heart disease), maybe you can ignore the medical warnings, learn to like your body as it is, and make yourself less crazy. On the other hand, if you have relevant health risks or feel that your weight interferes with the life you would like to lead, it is worth experimenting with lifestyle changes to find ways of losing weight gradually without dieting or feeling deprived.

• Think about what food means to you and the role eating plays in your life. Do you eat to satisfy hunger, to nourish your body, or do you eat to relieve anxiety, to try to fill up an inner emptiness? You can change your relationship to food if the latter two motives are the root of the problem, and you may need professional help to do so. Consider psychotherapy, visualization therapy, hypnotherapy, twelve-step programs, eating-disorder clinics, and other resources.

• Resolve to abandon crash dieting and ignore whatever weight-loss fad sweeps the country next. The solution to your problem is not there.

Diet

• Most people will lose weight if they take in fewer calories and increase the calories they burn through activity. Since fat has almost twice the number of calories per unit weight as carbohydrate and protein, the easiest place to begin is to identify the sources of fat in your diet and try to cut down. If, however, you simply replace fat with high-calorie simple carbohydrates—sugars and starches—you may not improve your situation and might even make it worse. As fat-free and low-fat versions of popular foods have come into widespread use in our country, obesity has steadily increased. Why? Probably because people are eating more calories. Fat-free cookies are not calorie-free, yet some people eat them in unlimited quantities. Pay attention to total calories, and replace high-fat foods with low-calorie foods like vegetables.

• Be aware of the glycemic index of common carbohydrate foods (see the table in the appendix). This is the measure of how easily the body turns them into glucose, provoking an insulin response. Table sugar has a glycemic index of 100. Values higher than that indicate strong potential to affect the insulin system, possibly predisposing you to weight gain; lower values indicate foods that you can eat more frequently and abundantly. There are surprises here: rice cakes, often thought of as diet food, have a very high glycemic index, both because of the chemical nature of the starch they contain and because of their "exploded" mechanical structure, which offers a greater surface area for digestive enzymes to work on; potatoes rank high also, as does bread, but whole-grain bread converts to sugar less rapidly than white bread, because the presence of fiber slows down the enzymatic process. Pasta ranks somewhat lower than bread, because its structure is more dense. If you have failed to lose weight on low-fat diets, insulin resistance may be your problem, in which case you want to moderate consumption of high-glycemic-index foods. People who develop insulin resistance usually have high serum triglycerides, gain weight easily, especially in the abdomen, and often crave carbohydrates. That does not mean anything is wrong with them; they just need to pay attention to the kinds and amounts of carbohydrate-rich foods they eat.

• Moderate or eliminate alcoholic beverages. The body treats alcohol as a high-glycemic-index carbohydrate. Its caloric energy cannot be stored but must be burned immediately, increasing the likelihood that the food you eat along with it will turn into fat.

• If you pay attention to the total calories you eat and increase your activity, the diet recommended in the Eight-Week Program should help you gradually move toward your ideal weight without thinking about it.

• Avoid artificial sweeteners and foods made with them. They will not help you lose weight and are hazardous to your health.

• Also avoid foods made with the new synthetic fat-substitutes. They may be unhealthy and will not help you change eating habits in the right manner.

• Try consulting a practitioner of Ayurvedic medicine or traditional Chinese medicine. Those systems emphasize finding the right way of eating to match your body type and might be able to provide you with helpful information about which foods to eat more of and which to avoid. People are different, and what works as a dietary plan for you may be different from what will work for me. Be willing to experiment and pay attention to the results.

Supplements

• Be skeptical of products in drug- and health-food stores that promise easy weight loss. Many contain stimulant drugs like ephedrine and phenylpropanolamine, or stimulant herbs like ephedra, guarana, and kola. Stimulants reduce appetite and speed up metabolism, and they also cause jitteriness, anxiety, insomnia, and drug dependence. When you stop taking them, weight will rapidly rebound. The prescription drugs in widespread use (fenfluramine and phentermine, sometimes called *fen-phen* when used in combination) are stronger but no different in kind, and no better with regard to long-term outcomes.

• Two currently popular weight-loss aids are chromium and garcinia. Supplemental chromium can affect the insulin system, because that mineral is needed by cells along with insulin to absorb glucose from the blood. Recently, high doses (1,000 micrograms daily) have been shown to normalize blood sugar in adult-onset diabetics, so chromium might ameliorate insulin resistance. Unfortunately, I know of no good evidence that it helps people lose weight. Garcinia is a fruit from Southeast Asia containing an unusual sour compound (HCA or hydroxycitric acid) that may block conversion of glucose to fat in the liver. It appears harmless, but reliable clinical data on its efficacy for weight loss in humans are nonexistent.

Exercise

• Exercise is critical in a successful program to normalize weight. It must be regular and vigorous enough to influence the appetite-regulating center in the brain as well as to burn up calories. Increase your activity any way you can and at every opportunity. Walking is fine for the purpose if you do enough of it (at least the minimum amounts called for in the program). Whatever you can do on top of that will help even more.

Mental/Spiritual

Obesity is as much a mental/spiritual problem as a physical one. I have known men and women who have dropped weight effortlessly and permanently after making changes in how they thought about themselves and perceived their bodies.

• If you eat to reduce anxiety or dull an inner sense of discomfort, try to use the Relaxing Breath to change this pattern. When you feel a craving for food unrelated to physical hunger, practice the Relaxing Breath before you act on it. By the time you finish, the craving may well have passed. This is a long-term project; keep at it.

• If you eat for emotional satisfaction or because you require oral stimulation, try to select foods that are lower in calories, fat, and high-glycemic-index carbohydrates. Most fruits and vegetables are safe choices.

• Practice liking your body as it is, because that is the only mind-set from which you can change it. As long as you do not accept and love your body, it will resist your desire to have it be different. I realize that loving an overweight body in a culture obsessed with thinness is difficult. Just keep working at it, and do not hesitate to call on professionals to help.

24

FOR THOSE AT RISK FOR CARDIOVASCULAR DISEASE

CARDIOVASCULAR DISEASE IS the number-one killer in our society, producing a great deal of disability as well as premature death, and absorbing countless health-care dollars. Its incidence rises sharply with age, affecting men earlier in life than women. Cardiovascular disease causes not only heart attacks and strokes (which might be better thought of as "brain attacks," because there are now emergency treatments for them that can be lifesaving if given with the same urgency as that with which we treat cardiac disasters) but also kidney failure, pain and gangrene in the lower extremities, and mental disability. The underlying disease process—arteriosclerosis (literally "hardening of the arteries")—damages arterial walls, making them inelastic, thick, and rough, eventually narrowing the channel within and decreasing blood flow. One component of this process is atherosclerosis, the deposition of fat and cholesterol in the walls of arteries, but the exact relationship between it and the larger disease is not clear. Arteriosclerosis is clearly a hazard of lifestyle, silent during its development, and of early onset in many people. Its prevention must be a high priority in any program designed to maintain optimum health.

It is clear that arteriosclerosis is multifactorial in origin. Among the contributing causes are heredity, diet, stress, lack of exercise, and toxins. The Eight-Week Program addresses all of these areas except heredity, of course, but in this customized plan I want to give you additional suggestions for prevention.

Projects

• Don't smoke, and don't inhale secondhand smoke. Nicotine directly affects arteries and is, in fact, one of the best-known toxins that accelerate arteriosclerosis; it is also a highly addictive drug. Besides nicotine, tobacco smoke contains other elements that undermine the health of arteries and many organs. If you smoke, set a date to quit, using any and all methods available to help you do so (see appendix). If you live or work with smokers, do whatever you can to get them to quit or confine their smoking to the outside. If those strategies fail, protect yourself with an air filter, as described in Week Four.
• Never drink water that tastes of chlorine. Order bottled water if you are out, and protect yourself at home with a water-purifying system. As a powerful oxidizing agent, chlorine is another common toxin that promotes arteriosclerosis.

Diet

Very recently, the homocysteine theory of arteriosclerosis, first proposed decades ago, has begun to gain support from medical researchers. In brief, it states that homocysteine, an amino acid produced by the metabolic breakdown of methionine, an essential component of dietary protein, is an independent risk factor for cardiovascular disease, one that may turn out to be more important than serum cholesterol. Animal protein delivers significantly more methionine than plant protein, which may explain why vegetarians are less likely to suffer from arteriosclerosis even though they eat more fat than some doctors think they should. The production and disposition of homocysteine are controlled by three B vitamins: pyridoxine (B_6), cyanocobalamin (B_{12}), and folic acid. Mainstream Western diets, with their overloads of animal protein and deficiencies of fresh fruits and vegetables, may fail to provide enough of these vitamins to handle the amounts of homocysteine generated and clear them from the blood. I am much impressed by this theory and the history of its rejection by the "cholesterol establishment"; I recommend watching for reports of experiments designed to confirm it.

• Tests for serum homocysteine are just becoming available. The normal value ranges around 10.0 micromoles per liter but must be adjusted for sex and age. If you have a family history of cardiovascular disease, ask your doctor to check your serum homocysteine.

• The dietary recommendations that follow from the homocysteine theory will be familiar to you from the Eight-Week Program. Note that they also may explain the effectiveness of the drastic diets that have been used to reverse atherosclerosis (fat reduction to 10 percent of calories or less, elimination of animal foods, and emphasis on fruits and vegetables). If homocysteine is really a major culprit, you may be able to relax about fat, enjoying the olive oil and salmon I recommend, and protecting yourself in other ways. Those ways are:

• Reducing animal protein in the diet as much as you can. Moderate consumption of fish is OK. In fact, since vitamin B_{12} comes only in nonplant foods, some fish (or nonfat or low-fat dairy products) is desirable.
• Eating plenty of fresh fruits and vegetables, including cooked greens, which are major sources of folic acid.
• Increasing consumption of dietary fiber by replacing refined grains with whole grains as much as possible: less white bread, more whole-grain bread; less white rice, more brown rice.
• Reducing consumption of white sugar and sweets in general. Diets high in sugar are most likely to be deficient in protective factors.
• Reducing consumption of packaged and highly processed foods, which are similarly deficient. A heart- and artery-healthy diet must emphasize fresh foods, always your best sources of vitamins and minerals.

• Include in your diet as many protective factors as you can that reduce risk of cardiovascular disease by other mechanisms: garlic, onions, hot peppers, green tea, shiitake mushrooms, salmon, and sardines (or flax). All of them improve serum-lipid profiles and help keep serum cholesterol in safe ranges.
• If you drink coffee, try to switch to tea, especially green tea, which is much better for the cardiovascular system. At least substitute green tea for some of the coffee you drink.
• Remember to enjoy your food! A diet that is healthy for the heart and arteries can also be diverse and delicious. If you make yourself miserable through deprivation, your spirits will suffer, and you will not be experiencing optimum health.

Supplements

• For insurance against elevated serum homocysteine, take a B-complex vitamin supplement every day. I recommend a B-100 brand. Read the label to make sure it provides 100 milligrams of vitamin B_6 and 400 micrograms of folic acid. (Note that one of the components of this supplement, vitamin B_2 or riboflavin, will color your urine bright yellow for a few hours, a harmless change.)

• Be sure to take the recommended dosage of antioxidants. More and more studies support the role of vitamin E in preventing atherosclerosis, probably by protecting LDL cholesterol from oxidation. Vitamin C may protect the integrity of arterial walls, reducing their susceptibility to damage by whatever injurious factors may be circulating in the blood.

• Follow a low-dose aspirin regimen to reduce the chance of abnormal blood-clotting. I recommend 162 milligrams a day—half of a standard tablet or two of the low-dose 81-milligram tablets.

• If you have any heart problems or a family history of them, take 100 milligrams a day of coenzyme Q (Co-Q-10), a natural product that increases oxygen utilization by heart-muscle cells. You will find this supplement in health-food stores; shop around for the best value and the highest dosage form you can find, so that you do not have to take more than one pill a day. (A side benefit of coenzyme Q is improved health of gums.)

• Do not take supplemental iron unless you have iron-deficiency anemia, diagnosed by blood tests. Iron is a risk factor for arteriosclerosis, by virtue of being an oxidizing agent that can increase oxidation of cholesterol into more harmful forms. Read labels of any multivitamin-and-mineral supplement you use to be sure it does not contain iron.

Exercise

• Do not neglect the exercise component of the Eight-Week Program. Regular aerobic exercise helps maintain normal weight and blood pressure, increases the efficiency of the heart as a pump, and preserves normal elasticity of arteries. It is a key preventive strategy to reduce the risk of cardiovascular disease. Walk!

Mental/Spiritual

• Stress raises serum cholesterol and blood pressure and renders the arteries more susceptible to spasms that can initiate heart and brain attacks. Practice techniques of stress reduction and relaxation, beginning with the Relaxing Breath.
• Learn to control toxic emotions, especially rage when frustrated, which appears to pose a particular risk for the cardiovascular system. Psychotherapy, counseling, group work, and relaxation training can all be helpful.
• Read over the sections of the program pertaining to connectedness and forgiveness. Try to implement them.
• Practice loving yourself whenever you can; this is the basis for being able to have loving relationships with others. Consider that the heart first pumps oxygen-rich blood to itself through the coronary arteries, then sends it to the rest of the body. If it did not do so, it would be unable to supply all the needs beyond it. Self-love is not selfishness or self-centeredness but the basis for extending love beyond yourself. Here is a version of the Buddhist meditation on *metta* (loving-kindness), which you can memorize and recite silently if it appeals to you, envisioning your love extending to each widening circle in turn. Note how it begins:

My heart fills with loving-kindness. I love myself. May I be happy.
   May I be peaceful. May I be liberated.
May all beings in this vicinity be happy. May they be happy. May they
   be liberated.
May all beings in [name your place of residence] *be happy. May they*
   be peaceful. May they be liberated.
May all beings in [name your state or region] *be happy. May they be*
   peaceful. May they be liberated.
May all beings in [name your country] *be happy. May they be peaceful. May they be liberated.*
May all beings in [name your continent] *be happy. May they be*
   peaceful. May they be liberated.
May all beings on the planet be happy. May they be peaceful. May
   they be liberated.

May my parents be happy. May they be well. May they be peaceful. May they be liberated.

May my friends be happy. May they be well. May they be peaceful. May they be liberated.

May my enemies be happy. May they be well. May they be peaceful. May they be liberated.

If I have hurt anyone, knowingly or unknowingly, in thought or word or deed, I ask their forgiveness.

If anyone has hurt me, knowingly or unknowingly, in thought or word or deed, I extend my forgiveness.

May all beings everywhere, whether near or far, whether known to me or unknown to me, be happy. May they be peaceful. May they be liberated.

Not a bad way to start the day. Give it a try.

25

FOR THOSE AT RISK FOR CANCER

WE SHOULD ALL PROBABLY consider ourselves at risk for cancer, since the incidence of that family of diseases is increasing in all age groups throughout the world. Therefore, I want to add some recommendations to the Eight-Week Program that are specifically intended to reduce cancer risk.

When I was a medical student in the late 1960s, the scientific establishment seemed reluctant to focus on environmental causes of cancer. Except for identifying cigarette smoke as the major risk factor for lung and bladder cancer and citing such historical examples as the high incidence of scrotal cancers among chimneysweeps in England, researchers looked to viral or genetic causes of the malignant transformation of cells. I was taught that diet was not a significant factor in cancer, in either its prevention or its treatment, and that anyone advocating vitamin or mineral supplements to reduce cancer risk was a quack.

This has all changed in the past few years. Experts at the National Cancer Institute now estimate that 35 percent of cancer deaths are attributable to diet alone, and the medical literature is full of recent studies demonstrating the preventive potential of specific foods and supplements. The scientific establishment is still reluctant to look at the contribution of agrichemicals, pesticides in particular, to the worldwide epidemic of cancer, but I predict that will change as well.

Cancer appears in the body for two reasons. First, a cell must undergo malignant transformation, removing it from normal controls on growth, longevity, and responsiveness to the needs of the whole organism. Second, a transformed cell must avoid identification and destruction by the body's defenses.

Malignant transformation results from genetic accident or the activity of tumor-inducing genes, viruses, and carcinogenic agents, either energetic (like X-rays) or material (like tobacco smoke). Biologists assume that malignant transformation occurs all the time, but that in almost all cases the body recognizes and eliminates the altered cells. Just how it does so is not clear. We know that the immune system's natural-killer (NK) cells are efficient destroyers of malignant cells, and a popular theory is that one of the principal functions of the immune system is constant surveillance of all tissues to look for transformed cells. There is a significant problem with this theory of immune surveillance, however: when the immune system is suppressed by drugs (as in organ-transplant recipients) or by disease (as in AIDS), we do not see a general increase in cancer. Instead, we see increased susceptibility to a limited number of cancers, such as certain leukemias, lymphomas, and skin cancers. People with transplanted kidneys and people with AIDS do not get more cancer of their lungs, prostates, breasts, or colons than the rest of us. If immune surveillance stands between malignant transformation and the development of cancer, why shouldn't knocking out the immune system lead to cancer throughout the body?

One possible answer is that the particular aspect of immunity responsible for identifying and eliminating transformed cells persists, despite suppression by drugs and viruses. Another answer is that the body has other methods to deal with malignancy. Cells throughout the body are genetically programmed to commit suicide if malignant transformation occurs, for example.

Even though scientists do not yet know just how cancers arise, I can tell you that the Eight-Week Program offers you great protection. Your best defense against malignant transformation is to avoid common carcinogens and bring protective factors into your life. Your best defense against the persistence of transformed cells in the body is to strive for optimum health, because the more you move toward that goal, the more efficiently all of the defensive functions of your healing system will perform.

Projects

• Look over your family history and identify the frequency and types of cancer that have occurred. This information can pinpoint those areas of lifestyle of greatest concern.

• Know the early warning signs of cancer (see appendix) and the common screening tests (such as Pap smears for women and serum-PSA tests for men) that can identify cancers that are easily curable in their earliest stages.

• Do not smoke and do not inhale secondhand smoke. Tobacco smoke is the most important environmental cause of cancer (and tobacco addiction is the most common preventable cause of serious disease in the world).

• Do not drink alcohol immoderately. Heavy drinkers are more likely than others to develop cancers of the mouth, throat, esophagus, stomach, and liver (and are at even greater risk if they also smoke). Drink moderately, minimally, or not all. If you are female, pay attention to new information about the hazards of moderate intake of alcohol, which may increase risk of breast cancer in genetically susceptible individuals by way of its influence on the body's production and distribution of estrogen.

• Follow all of the suggestions in the program for minimizing your exposure to toxins in water, air, and food.

• Inform yourself about harmful forms of radiation and chemicals, and take steps to limit your exposure to them. (See appendix.)

Diet

• Avoid carcinogenic foods. Black pepper, button mushrooms (the common cultivated variety), peanuts, and peanut products all contain natural carcinogens, so limit intake of them. Celery and raw legume sprouts (alfalfa sprouts in particular) contain natural toxins that harm the immune system. In addition, heavily salted and smoked foods and types of pickles used in Asia (aged radishes and turnips, for example) are carcinogenic when consumed regularly, as are barbecued meats or any animal foods cooked until the surface is blackened. (If you have to eat these, cut away the blackened outer portion.) Reduce or eliminate cured meats—ones that look red because they have been treated with nitrite preservatives. Avoid artificially colored foods and all artificial sweeteners.

• Eat a high-fiber diet to protect against colorectal cancer, breast cancer, and, possibly, other hormonally driven cancers. That means more whole-grain products instead of refined ones.

• Eat plenty of fresh fruits and vegetables. By doing so, you will get the chemopreventive benefits of sulphoraphane and other indoles in broccoli, lycopene in tomatoes, limonene in citrus fruits, ellagic acid in grapes and apples, carotenoids in all the yellow and orange fruits and vegetables as well as in leafy greens, isoflavones in soybeans, and many other factors yet to be identified. Don't forget the garlic and ginger.

Supplements

• Make the antioxidant formula an ongoing part of your life. It offers great benefits, both by helping your body neutralize carcinogens and by protecting its abilities to recognize and eliminate malignant cells.

• If you have a family history of cancer, have been a smoker, have worked in a hazardous occupation, or know that you have had toxic exposures, take one or more of the tonics that are cancer-protective and immune-enhancing. (Review the information on tonics in Week Six.) My first choices would be maitake and reishi mushrooms. Astragalus is another possibility. I also recommend a low-dose aspirin regimen—162 milligrams a day—since aspirin reduces risk of esophageal and colon cancer.

Exercise

• By virtue of its central role in fostering optimum health, regular exercise also helps protect you from cancer. Do it.

Mental/Spiritual

• Although much is in print about cancer-prone personalities, I am unconvinced that medical science has demonstrated any links between personality types and cancer risks. Nonetheless, it is obvious to me that grief and depression impair resistance and health in general, so I would not be surprised to learn that mental and spiritual imbalances make people more susceptible to cancer. Working to improve mental/spiritual health by means of the techniques suggested in the program cannot fail to bolster defenses against all kinds of disease, including cancer.

Appendix

Finding Information
and Supplies

FLAXSEEDS AND GRINDERS

Heintzman Farms
RR2, Box 265
Onaka, SD 57466
800 333-5813

VITAMIN C

C-Salts (effervescent, nonacidic
powder)
Wholesale Nutrition
P.O. Box 3345
Saratoga, CA 95070-9942
800 325-2664

PORTABLE CARBON
WATER FILTERS

Magellan's Catalogue
Box 5485
Santa Barbara, CA 93150-5485
800 962-4943

H2O International Inc.
3001 Southwest 15th Street, Suite B
Deerfield Beach, FL 33442
800 955-8561

LABORATORIES FOR TESTING
DRINKING WATER

National Testing Laboratories
6555 Wilson Mills Road
Cleveland, OH 44143
800 458-3330

Spectrum Labs
301 West County Road E2
St. Paul, MN 55112
612 633-0101

INFORMATION ON WATER
PURIFIERS

National Sanitation Foundation (NSF)
3475 Plymouth Road
Ann Arbor, MI 48105
800 673-8010

Don't Drink the Water (1996) by
Lono Kahuna Kapua A'o
Kali Press
P.O. Box 2169
Pagosa Springs, CO 81147
970 264-5200

The Drinking Water Book (1996) by
Colin Ingram
Ten Speed Press
P.O. Box 7123
Berkeley, CA 94707
800 841-2665

INFORMATION ON ORGANIC PRODUCE

Mothers & Others for a Livable Planet
40 West 20th Street
New York, NY 10011
212 242-0010

Environmental Working Group
1718 Connecticut Avenue, N.W.,
Suite 600
Washington, DC 20009
202 667-6982

Eden Acres, Inc.
12100 Lima Center Road
Clinton, MI 49236
517 456-4288

ADJUSTABLE AIR MATTRESSES

Select Comfort Corporation
6150 Trenton Lane North
Minneapolis, MN 55442
800 831-1211

INFORMATION ON TOXIC ENERGY

Cross Currents: The Perils of Electro-pollution, The Promise of Electro-medicine, by Robert O. Becker, M.D.
(Los Angeles: Jeremy Tarcher, 1991).

SUN-PROTECTIVE FABRIC

Solumbra, made by Sun Precautions
2815 Wetmore Avenue
Everett, WA 98201
800 882-7860

STRETCHING

Stretching, Inc.
P.O. Box 767
Palmer Lake, CO 80133
800 333-1307

(distributors of books, videos, and equipment, including Stretching *by Bob Anderson, the best book on the subject)*

OSTEOPATHIC MANIPULATIVE THERAPY

American Academy of Osteopathy
3500 De Pauw Boulevard, Suite 1080
Indianapolis, IN 46268
317 879-1881

CORDYCEPS AND OTHER TONIC MUSHROOMS

Fungi Perfecti
P.O. Box 7634
Olympia, WA 98507
800 780-9126
www.fungi.com

MAITAKE MUSHROOMS AND D-FRACTION

Maitake Products, Inc.
222 Bergen Turnpike
Ridgefield, NJ 07660
800 747-7418

ALTERNATIVES TO PRESCRIPTION DRUGS

Natural Alternatives to Over-the-Counter and Prescription Drugs, by Michael T. Murray (New York: William Morrow, 1994).

RESOURCES FOR WOMEN'S HEALTH

National Women's Health Network
(newsletter, information service)
514 10th Street, N.W., Suite 400
Washington, DC 20004
202 347-1140

National Women's Health Resource Center (information packets)
2425 L Street, N.W., Third Floor
Washington, DC 20037
202 293-6045

Harvard Women's Health Watch (monthly newsletter)
P.O. Box 420234
Palm Coast, FL 33142-0234
800 829-5921

Dr. Christiane Northrup's Health Wisdom for Women (monthly newsletter)
7811 Montrose Road
Potomac, MD 20854
301 424-3700

Dr. Andrew Weil's Self Healing (monthly newsletter)
42 Pleasant Street
Watertown, MA 02172
800 523-3296

The PDR (R) Family Guide to Women's Health and Prescription Drugs (Montvale, N.J.: Medical Economics, 1994).

Women's Health Companion: Self-Help Nutrition and Cookbook, by Susan Lark, M.D. (Berkeley, Calif.: Celestial Arts, 1995).

INFORMATION ON HORMONE-REPLACEMENT THERAPY FOR WOMEN

The Estrogen Decision, by Susan Lark, M.D. (Los Altos, Calif.: Westchester Publishing, 1994).

Estrogen: Is It Right for You?, by Paula Dranov (New York: Fireside, 1993).

The Menopause Industry, by Sandra Coney (Alameda, Calif.: Hunter House, 1994).

Women's Bodies, Women's Wisdom, by Christiane Northrup, M.D. (New York: Bantam, 1994).

INFORMATION ON TOUCH HEALING

Therapeutic Touch, by Dolores Krieger (Englewood Cliffs, N.J.: Prentice-Hall, 1979).

Hands of Light: A Guide to Healing Through the Human Energy Field, by Barbara Ann Brennan (New York: Bantam, 1988).

Bonnie Prudden
7800 East Speedway
Tucson, AZ 85710-1649
520 529-3979
800 221-4634

Jin Shin Jyutsu, Inc.
8219 East San Alberto
Scottsdale, AZ 85258
602 998-9331

The Center for Reiki Training
29209 Northwestern Highway, #592
Southfield, MI 48034
810 948-8112
www.reiki.org

WRIST BANDS FOR NAUSEA

Travel-Eze, available at drug stores

Morning Sickness Bands
Magellan's Catalogue
Box 5485
Santa Barbara, CA 93150-5485
800 962-4943

American Society of Clinical Hypnosis
2200 East Devon Avenue, Suite 291
Des Plaines, IL 60018
847 297-3317

Academy for Guided Imagery
P.O. Box 2070
Mill Valley, CA 94942
415 389-9324

ALTERNATIVE TREATMENTS FOR
CHILDHOOD AILMENTS

*The Holistic Pediatrician: A Parents'
Comprehensive Guide to Safe and
Effective Therapies for the Twenty-
Five Most Common Childhood Ail-
ments,* by Kathi J. Kemper, M.D.
(San Francisco: HarperCollins, 1996).

American Association of Naturo-
pathic Physicians
2366 Eastlake Avenue East, Suite 322
Seattle, WA 98102
206 323-7610

INFORMATION ON HEALTH
RISKS OF FLYING

Healthy Flying
P.O. Box 999
Hana, HI 96713
808 248-7700
diana@maui.net

RESOURCES FOR
WEIGHT CONTROL

TOPS Club, Inc. (Take Off Pounds
Sensibly)
P.O. Box 07360
Milwaukee, WI 53207
414 482-4620

Overeaters Anonymous
P.O. Box 92870
Los Angeles, CA 90069
213 542-8363

American Society of Bariatric
Physicians
5600 South Quebec, Suite 109A
Englewood, CO 80111
303 779-4833

GLYCEMIC-INDEX RATINGS OF
CARBOHYDRATE FOODS

Foods with a glycemic index of 100 or
above are very quick to release sugar
into the bloodstream. To slow down
this release, combine any food that
has a high glycemic index with another that has a low one.

Puffed rice	133
Rice cake	133
Corn flakes	121
Sugar	100
Bread	100
Baked potatoes	98
Carrots	92
Rice	82
Corn	82
Bananas	82
Raisins	64
Spaghetti	60
Pinto beans	60
Sweet potatoes	51
Oatmeal	49
Orange juice	46
Navy beans	40
Apples	39
Peaches	29
Plums	25
Fructose	20

METHODS TO QUIT SMOKING

The No-Nag, No-Guilt, Do-It-Your-

Own-Way Guide to Quitting Smoking, by Tom Ferguson, M.D. (New York: Ballantine, 1988).

Nicotine Anonymous World Services (twelve-step program)
2118 Greenwich Street
San Francisco, CA 94123
415 750-0328

American Lung Association (Freedom-from-Smoking materials)
1726 M Street, N.W., Suite 902
Washington, DC 20036-4502
800 586-4872
www.lungusa.org

WARNING SIGNS OF CANCER

- Change in bowel or bladder habits
- A sore that does not heal
- Obvious change in a wart or mole
- Unusual bleeding or discharge
- Thickening or lump in a breast or elsewhere
- Persistent indigestion or difficulty swallowing
- Persistent cough or hoarseness
- Unexplained loss of weight

American Cancer Society
1599 Clifton Road
Atlanta, GA 30329
800 227-2345
www.cancer.org

INFORMATION ON HARMFUL
FORMS OF RADIATION
AND CHEMICALS

Natural Health, Natural Medicine, by Andrew Weil, M.D. (Boston: Houghton Mifflin, 1995), pp. 171–200.

Raising Children Toxic Free, by Herbert Needleman, M.D, and Philip Landrigan, M.D. (New York: Farrar, Straus and Giroux, 1994).

Everyday Cancer Risks and How to Avoid Them, by Mary Kerney Levenstein (Garden City Park, N.Y.: Avery Publishing, 1992).

Radiation and Human Health, by John W. Gofman (San Francisco: Sierra Club Books, 1981).

Detailed instructions for management of common medical conditions with natural remedies that take advantage of the body's healing system will be found in my book *Natural Health, Natural Medicine.*

You may visit me on the World Wide Web at *Ask Dr. Weil,*
http://www.dr.weil.com/

If you would like information on my lectures and informational products, including my monthly newsletter, *Self Healing,* please write to:

Andrew Weil, M.D.
P.O. Box 457
Vail, AZ 85641

NOTES

PART ONE: THE CAPACITY TO CHANGE

1. People Can Change

4   my first book: Andrew Weil, *The Natural Mind: A New Way of Looking at Drugs and the Higher Consciousness* (Boston: Houghton Mifflin, 1972).

5   written elsewhere about those travels: Andrew Weil, *The Marriage of the Sun and Moon: A Quest for Unity in Consciousness* (Boston: Houghton Mifflin, 1980).

I describe seeking out a shaman: Andrew Weil, *Spontaneous Healing: How to Discover and Enhance Your Body's Natural Ability to Maintain and Heal Itself* (New York: Alfred A. Knopf, 1995), pp. 11–19.

2. An Overview of Health and Healing

15 *Ganoderma* increases immune destruction: E. Furesawa et al., "Antitumor Activity of *Ganoderma lucidum* on Intraperitoneally Implanted Lewis Lung Carcinoma in Syngenic Mice," *Phytotherapy Research,* vol. 6 (1992), pp. 300–304.

16 Jordan Houghton: R. Hirschhorn et al., "Spontaneous In Vivo Reversion to Normal of an Inherited Mutation in a Patient with Adenosine Deaminase Deficiency," *Nature Genetics,* vol. 13 (1996), pp. 290–95.

17 "Suppose I come down . . .": Weil, *Spontaneous Healing,* p. 110.

3. The Whole Picture

25 emotional risk factors for heart attacks: W. Jiang et al., "Mental Stress-Induced Myocardial Ischemia and Cardiac Events," *Journal of the American Medical Association,* vol. 275 (1996), pp. 1651–56.

27   vitamin-C deficiency and coronary heart disease: M. Rath and L. Pauling,
     "Hypothesis: Lipoprotein(a) is a surrogate for ascorbate," *Proceedings of
     the National Academy of Sciences,* vol. 87 (1990), pp. 6204–7; M. Rath
     and L. Pauling, "Immunological Evidence for the Accumulation of
     Lipoprotein(a) in the Atherosclerotic Lesion of the Hypoascorbemic
     Guinea Pig," *Proceedings of the National Academy of Sciences,* vol. 87
     (1990), pp. 9388–90.

28   associate emotions with the heart: J. C. Barefoot and M. Schroll, "Symp-
     toms of Depression, Acute Myocardial Infarction, and Total Mortality in
     a Community Sample," *Circulation,* vol. 93 (1996), pp. 1976–80; P.
     Gunby, "Medical News & Perspectives: Depression and the Heart," *Jour-
     nal of the American Medical Association,* vol. 276 (1996), p. 1123.

4. Why Eight Weeks?

35   On adverse effects of NSAIDs, see C. E. Cooke, "Disease Management:
     Prevention of NSAID-Induced Gastropathy," *Drug Benefit Trends,* vol. 8
     (1996), pp. 14–15, 19–22.

36   well-known studies of hypnosis: L. F. Chapman et al., "Changes in Tissue
     Vulnerability Induced by Hypnotic Suggestion," *American Journal of
     Clinical Hypnosis,* vol. 2 (1960), p. 172.

38   Licorice builds up the mucous coating: K. D. Bardhan et al., "Clinical Trial
     of Deglycyrrhizinated Liquorice in Gastric Ulcer," *Gut,* vol. 19 (1978), pp.
     779–82; A. G. Morgan et al., "Comparison Between Cimetidine and
     Caved-S in the Treatment of Gastric Ulceration, and Subsequent Mainte-
     nance Therapy," *Gut,* vol. 23 (1982), pp. 545–51.

PART TWO: THE EIGHT-WEEK PROGRAM

5. Week One

49   *trans*-fatty acids: "Special Task Force Report: Position Paper on Trans
     Fatty Acids 1–3," *American Journal of Clinical Nutrition,* vol. 63 (1996),
     pp. 663–70; W. C. Willett, "Diet and Health: What Should We Eat," *Sci-
     ence,* vol. 264 (1994), pp. 532–37.

50   artificial, noncaloric sweeteners: R. G. Walton et al., "Adverse Reactions
     to Aspartame: Double-Blind Challenge in Patients from a Vulnerable Pop-
     ulation," *Biological Psychiatry,* vol. 34 (1993), pp. 13–17; S. K. Van den
     Eeden et al., "Aspartame Ingestion and Headaches: A Randomized
     Crossover Trial," *Neurology,* vol. 44 (1994), pp. 1787–93; D. Wein, "Are
     Artificial Sweeteners Safe? EN Updates a Sticky Issue," *Environmental
     Nutrition,* vol. 18 (1995), pp. 1–2.

51 On the health benefits of fish, see T. A. Mori et al., "Effects of Varying Dietary Fat, Fish, and Fish Oils on Blood Lipids in a Randomized Controlled Trial in Men at Risk of Heart Disease," *American Journal of Clinical Nutrition,* vol. 59 (1994), pp. 1060–69; P. Pauletto, "Blood Pressure and Atherogenic Lipoprotein Profiles in Fish-Diet and Vegetarian Villagers in Tanzania: The Lugalawa Study," *Lancet,* vol. 348 (1996), pp. 784–88.

60 I have written extensively about the healing power of breath: Andrew Weil, *Natural Health, Natural Medicine* (Boston: Houghton Mifflin, 1995), pp. 85–92, 119–20; Weil, *Spontaneous Healing,* pp. 203–7.

6. Week Two

65 On the dangers of nitrates in drinking water, see M. H. Ward et al., "Drinking Water Nitrate and the Risk of Non-Hodgkin's Lymphoma," *Epidemiology,* vol. 7 (1996), pp. 465–71.

69 On environmental xenoestrogens, see Theo Colborn, Dianne Dumanoski, and John Peterson Myers, *Our Stolen Future: Are We Threatening Our Fertility, Intelligence, and Survival? A Scientific Detective Story* (New York: Dutton, 1996); John Wargo, *Our Children's Toxic Legacy: How Science and Law Fail to Protect Us from Pesticides* (New Haven, Conn.: Yale University Press, 1996).

71 health benefits of green tea: H. N. Graham, "Green Tea Composition, Consumption, and Polyphenol Chemistry," *Preventive Medicine,* vol. 21 (1992), pp. 334–50; K. Imai and K. Nakachi, "Cross Sectional Study of Effects of Drinking Green Tea on Cardiovascular and Liver Diseases," *British Medical Journal,* vol. 310 (1995), pp. 693–96; W. Zheng et al., "Tea Consumption and Cancer Incidence in a Prospective Cohort Study of Postmenopausal Women," *American Journal of Epidemiology,* vol. 144 (1996), pp. 175–82.

77 new research on beta-carotene: C. Marwick, "Trials Reveal No Benefit, Possible Harm of Beta Carotene and Vitamin A for Lung Cancer Prevention," *Journal of the American Medical Association,* vol. 275 (1996), pp. 422–23; "Beta-Carotene: Helpful or Harmful?," *Science,* vol. 264 (1994), p. 500.
On lycopene and prostate cancer, see E. Giovannucci et al., "Intake of Carotenoids and Retinol in Relation to Risk of Prostate Cancer," *Journal of the National Cancer Institute,* vol. 87 (1995), pp. 1767–76.

79 I have written elsewhere about visualization: Weil, *Spontaneous Healing,* pp. 93–97, 199–201.

7. Week Three

85 An experiment reported: S. Arnold et al., "Synergistic Activation of Estrogen Receptor with Combinations of Environmental Chemicals," *Science,*

vol. 272 (1996), pp. 1489–92; S. Simons, "Environmental Estrogens: Can Two 'Alrights' Make a Wrong?," *Science,* vol. 272 (1996), p. 1451.

86   I have written elsewhere about the hazards of ionizing radiation: Weil, *Natural Health, Natural Medicine,* pp. 174–78.

87   On health hazards of electromagnetic fields, see Robert O. Becker, *Cross Currents: The Perils of Electropollution, The Promise of Electromedicine* (Los Angeles: Jeremy Tarcher, 1991); P. Coogan et al., "Occupational Exposure to 60-Hertz Magnetic Fields and Risk of Breast Cancer in Women," *Epidemiology,* vol. 7 (1996), pp. 459–64; K. A. Fackelmann, "Do EMFs Pose Breast Cancer Risk (Exposure to Low-Frequency Electromagnetic Fields)?," *Science News,* vol. 145 (1994), p. 388.

8. Week Four

103   house plants that absorb toxic gases from the air: J. Barilla, "Natural Filters That Trap Air Pollution Without Energy Cost and Look Nice Too," *Health News and Review,* Winter 1995, p. 15; "The Hidden Life of Spider Plants," *University of California at Berkeley Wellness Letter,* vol. 10 (February 1994), p. 1.

104   health benefits of garlic: Heinrich P. Koch and Larry D. Lawson, *Garlic: The Science and Therapeutic Application of* Allium sativum *L. and Related Species,* 2nd ed. (Baltimore: Williams & Wilkins, 1996).

9. Week Five

114   the Native American sweat lodge: Weil, *Marriage of Sun and Moon,* pp. 247–52.

115   "For the Finns . . .": Tom Johnson and Tim Miller, *The Sauna Book* (New York: Harper & Row, 1977), p. 3.

117   remarkable therapeutic effects of ginger: Paul Schulick, *Ginger: Common Spice & Wonder Drug,* rev. ed. (Brattleboro, Vt.: Herbal Free Press, 1994).

10. Week Six

132   We now know that ginseng: S. Shibata et al., "Chemistry and Pharmacology of Panax," *Economic and Medicinal Plant Research,* vol. 1 (1985), pp. 217–84; L. D'Angelo et al., "A Double-Blind, Placebo-Controlled Clinical Study on the Effect of a Standardized Ginseng Extract on Psychomotor Performance in Healthy Volunteers," *Journal of Ethnopharmacology,* vol. 16 (1986), pp. 15–22.

133   On the health benefits of aspirin, see L. Marnett, "Aspirin and the Role of Prostaglandins in Cancer," *Cancer Research,* vol. 52 (1992), pp. 5575–89; M. Thun et al., "Aspirin Use and Risk of Fatal Cancer," *Cancer Research,*

vol. 53 (1993), pp. 1322–27; R. Rozzini et al., "Protective Effect of Chronic NSAID Use on Cognitive Decline in Older Persons," *Journal of the American Geriatrics Society,* vol. 44 (1996), pp. 1025–29.

134 On the effects of ashwagandha, see M. Ziauddin et al., "Studies on the Immunomodulatory Effects of Ashwagandha," *Journal of Ethnopharmacology,* vol. 50 (1996), pp. 69–76.

Recent animal research: A. Grandhi et al., "A Comparative Pharmacological Investigation of Ashwagandha and Ginseng," *Journal of Ethnopharmacology,* vol. 44 (1994), pp. 131–35.

On the effects of astragalus, see "Astragalus" in A. Y. Leung and S. Foster, *Encyclopedia of Common Natural Ingredients* (New York: John Wiley & Sons, 1995).

135 On the effects of cordyceps, see A. Tsunoo, "*Cordyceps sinensis:* Its Diverse Effects on Mammals in vitro and in vivo," *New Initiatives in Mycological Research* (proceedings of the third International Symposium of the Mycological Society of Japan), Chiba, Japan: Natural History Museum and Institute, Chiba, 1995.

136 On the effects of dong quai, see James A. Duke and Edward S. Ayensu, *Medicinal Plants of China* (Algonac, Mich.: Reference Publications, 1985), pp. 74–77; K. Yoshiro, "The Physiological Actions of Tang-Kuei and Cnidium," *Bulletin of the Oriental Healing Arts Institute USA,* vol. 10 (1985), pp. 269–78.

137 On the benefits of maitake, see H. Nanba, "Activity of Maitake D-Fraction to Inhibit Carcinogenesis and Metastasis," *Annals of the New York Academy of Sciences,* vol. 768 (1995), pp. 243–45.

138 On the effects of milk thistle, see V. Fintelmann and A. Albert, *Therapiewoche,* vol. 30 (1980), pp. 5589–94; H. Hikino and Y. Kiso, "Natural Products for Liver Disease," in H. Wagner, H. Hikino, and N. R. Farnsworth, eds., *Economic and Medicinal Plant Research,* vol. 2 (New York: Academic Press, 1988), pp. 39–72.

On the effects of reishi, see J. Lin et al., "Radical Scavenger and Antihepatotoxic Activity of *Ganoderma formosanum, Ganoderma lucidum,* and *Ganoderma neo-japonicum,*" *Journal of Ethnopharmacology,* vol. 47 (1995), pp. 33–41.

139 On the effects of Siberian ginseng: N. R. Farnsworth et al., "Siberian Ginseng (*Eleutherococcus senticosus*): Current Status as an Adaptogen," in H. Wagner, H. Hikino, and N. R. Farnsworth, eds., *Economic and Medicinal Plant Research,* vol. 1 (Orlando, Fla.: Academic Press, 1985), pp. 155–215.

11. Week Seven

160 "Begin by slowly bringing . . .": Stephen Levine, *Healing into Life and Death* (New York: Doubleday, 1987), p. 98.

12. Week Eight

166 "Use meat as a side dish . . .": *The New York Times,* September 17, 1996, p. A16.
169 what I have written about the effects of coffee: Weil, *Natural Health, Natural Medicine,* pp. 140–44.
172 the way we experience reality is influenced by concepts: See my books *The Natural Mind* and *Marriage of Sun and Moon,* as well as the four-leaf-clover story in *Spontaneous Healing,* pp. 195–96.

PART THREE: THE CUSTOMIZED PLANS

15. For Those over Age Seventy

198 "When I was only 19 . . .": Thich Nhat Hanh, *The Miracle of Mindfulness: A Manual on Meditation,* trans. Mobi Ho (Boston: Beacon Press, rev. ed. 1976), p. 50.
199 On the effects of ginkgo, see J. Kleijnen and P. Knipschild, "*Ginkgo biloba* for Cerebral Insufficiency," *British Journal of Clinical Pharmacology,* vol. 34 (1992), pp. 352–58.
200 "Lie on a bed . . .": Thich Nhat Hanh, *Miracle of Mindfulness,* p. 90.

17. For Men

208 saw palmetto: G. Champault et al., "A Double-Blind Trial of an Extract of the Plant *Serenoa repens* in Benign Prostatic Hyperplasia," *British Journal of Clinical Pharmacology,* vol. 18 (1984), pp. 461–62.

19. For Pregnant Women (and Those Considering Pregnancy)

215 "conscious conception and birth": Laura Archera Huxley and Piero Ferrucci, *The Child of Your Dreams* (Minneapolis: CompCare Publishers, 1987).
216 morning sickness as a protective reaction: Margie Profet, *Protecting Your Baby-to-Be* (Reading, Mass.: Addison-Wesley, 1995).
218 I told the story of my wife, Sabine: Weil, *Spontaneous Healing,* p. 97.

22. For Those Who Travel Frequently

230 The air quality in planes is dreadful: D. Fairchild, "Is Airplane Air Really Unhealthy and Germ Filled?" (1996), available from *Healthy Flying,* Box 999, Hana, HI 96713; 808 248-7700.

231 On the effects of echinacea, see B. Bräunig et al., "Echinacea Purpureae Radix for Strengthening the Immune Response in Flu-like Infections," *Zeitschrift für Phytotherapie,* vol. 13 (1992), pp. 7–13.

23. For Those Who Are Overweight

238 the glycemic index of foods: the information in the text and the table in the appendix are derived from K. Foster-Powell and J. B. Miller, "International Tables of Glycemic Index," *American Journal of Clinical Nutrition,* vol. 62 (1995), pp. 871S–93S.

239 On high doses of chromium in adult-onset diabetes, see R. Anderson, "Beneficial Effects of Chromium for People with Type II Diabetes," *Diabetes,* vol. 45 (1996), suppl. 2.

24. For Those at Risk for Cardiovascular Disease

242 the homocysteine theory of arteriosclerosis: Kilmer McCully, *The Homocysteine Revolution* (New Canaan, Conn.: Keats Publishing, 1997); O. Nygard et al., "Total Plasma Homocysteine and Cardiovascular Risk Profile—the Hordaland Homocysteine Study," *Journal of the American Medical Association,* vol. 274 (1995), pp. 1526–33.

244 On the benefits of coenzyme Q, see T. Kawasaki, "Antioxidant Function of Coenzyme Q," *Journal of Nutritional Science and Vitaminology,* vol. 38 (1992), spec. no., pp. 552–55.

25. For Those at Risk for Cancer

247 National Cancer Institute estimate: P. Greenwald et al., "New Directions in Dietary Studies in Cancer: The National Cancer Institute," in J. B. Longenecker et al., eds., *Nutrition and Biotechnology in Heart Disease and Cancer* (New York: Plenum Press, 1995), pp. 229–39.

249 alcohol may increase risk of breast cancer: M. P. Longnecker et al., "Risk of Breast Cancer in Relation to Lifetime Alcohol Consumption," *Journal of the National Cancer Institute,* vol. 87 (1995), pp. 923–29.

ACKNOWLEDGMENTS

Sonny Mehta, editor-in-chief of Alfred A. Knopf, asked me to write this book to fill a need created by my preceding work, *Spontaneous Healing*. I am grateful to him for the suggestion, and to my editor, Jonathan Segal, for his devotion to the task of making the text letter-perfect. I also thank Paul Bogaards, Jane Friedman, Carol Janeway, Ida Giragossian, and others at Knopf who helped bring this book from the realm of idea to that of manifestation in paper and ink.

My agent, Richard Pine, of Arthur Pine Associates, continues to be a trusted friend and supporter. Without his direction, my recent writings on health and healing would not have found such wide readership.

Persons who contributed information to this book include Paul Stamets, Ken Rosen, Jodie Evans, and Dr. Seymour Reichlin. Kim Cliffton and Nora Pouillon helped me get the recipes in order. Hannah Fisher at the reference desk of the University of Arizona Health Sciences Library looked up many journal citations for me. And I thank all of the patients and readers who sent me personal accounts of their experiences with healing and lifestyle change, some of which I've called upon here.

My wife, Sabine, as usual, ran both home and office while I was writing, and made it possible for me to have the time and space to complete the project. She also helped read and organize all of the letters that came from people who have followed my recommendations for self-healing. Our children, Robyn, Martin, Logan, and Diana, also helped, as did B.T., Jeep, Winnie, Kelty, and Jambo.

Lynn Willeford collected a great deal of information for the reference notes and appendix and made sure that my statements were consistent with scientific research. I thank Andrew Ungerleider and Gay Dillingham for their generous support, as well as the video-production team they helped organize: Sandra Hay, Pat Faust, and Tony Greco, especially. I also thank the members of the BOTS club for their attention and support: Fred Runkel, Chris Hall, Michael Meyer, Keith McDaniel, Ken Baker, Dr. Brian Becker, and Michael Peters.

Andrew Weil
Tucson, Arizona
January 1997

INDEX

Andrew Weil, M.D., a graduate of Harvard College and Harvard Medical School, worked for the National Institute of Mental Health and for fifteen years was a research associate in ethnopharmacology at the Harvard Botanical Museum. As a fellow of the Institute of Current World Affairs, he traveled extensively throughout the world collecting information about medicinal plants and healing. He is the founder of the Center for Integrative Medicine in Tucson, Arizona, and director of the Program in Integrative Medicine at the University of Arizona. This is Dr. Weil's seventh book.

A NOTE ON THE TYPE

The text of this book was set in Sabon, a typeface designed by Jan Tschichold (1902–1974), the well-known German typographer. Based loosely on the original designs by Claude Garamond (c. 1480–1561), Sabon is unique in that it was explicitly designed for hot metal composition on both the Monotype and Linotype machines as well as for filmsetting. Designed in 1966 in Frankfurt, Sabon was named for the famous Lyons punch cutter Jacques Sabon, who is thought to have brought some of Garamond's matrices to Frankfurt.

Composed by North Market Street Graphics, Lancaster, Pennsylvania.
Printed and bound by R. R. Donnelley & Sons, Harrisonburg, Virgina.